STOMACH ULCER DIET COOKBOOK

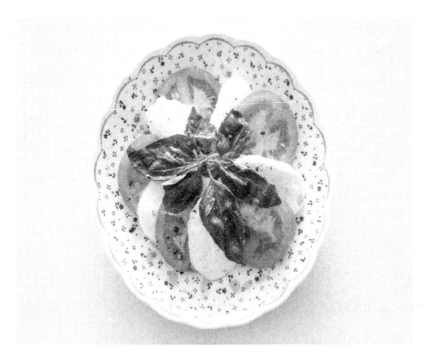

"Wholesome Recipes for Healing: A Stomach Ulcer Diet Cookbook"

FIONA L. BRYAN

TABLE OF CONTENT

INTRODUCTION

Once upon a time in the peaceful village of Greenwood, there lived a young woman named Blossom. She was known throughout the village for her radiant smile, boundless energy, and her unmatched talent in gardening. Blossom's garden was a marvel to behold. It was filled with vibrant flowers of every hue and aromatic herbs that seemed to dance in the breeze.

However, there was a secret that Blossom kept hidden from everyone. For the past few years, she had been suffering silently from a persistent and painful stomach ulcer. It had become so severe that she often found herself unable to enjoy the delicious fruits and vegetables she grew in her garden. The constant pain and discomfort left her feeling weak and tired, but she refused to give in to despair.

One day, while tending to her garden, Blossom noticed a small, brightly colored flower that she had never seen before. Its petals were a striking shade of violet, and it seemed to radiate a soothing energy. Curiosity piqued, she carefully examined the flower and discovered that it was called "Healing Blossom," known for its therapeutic properties.

Blossom decided to research the Healing Blossom and its potential benefits for her stomach ulcer. She delved into ancient herbology books, consulted with wise villagers, and experimented with different concoctions. After much trial and error, she crafted a tea using Healing Blossom petals, along with other stomach-soothing herbs from her garden.

She began drinking this special tea daily, and as the weeks passed, she noticed a gradual improvement in her health. The excruciating pain subsided, and her energy returned. Blossom's appetite improved, and she could once again savor the flavors of her own garden-fresh produce.

Word of Blossom's miraculous recovery began to spread throughout Greenwood. Villagers who suffered from various ailments sought her guidance, and she willingly shared her knowledge and her Healing Blossom tea recipe with them. Together, they planted Healing Blossom plants in their gardens, and the entire village experienced a newfound sense of well-being.

As Blossom's garden flourished and her reputation as a healer grew, she realized that her journey to recovery had a purpose greater than herself. She continued to study herbs and their healing properties, eventually becoming the village's trusted herbalist.

Years passed, and Blossom's legacy lived on. Her Healing Blossom tea became renowned far and wide, curing stomach ulcers and bringing comfort to many. Blossom's garden, once a personal sanctuary, had transformed into a place of healing and hope for the entire village.

Blossom's story served as a reminder that sometimes, the solutions to life's challenges can be found in the most unexpected places, and that the strength of the human spirit, combined with nature's gifts, can lead to remarkable transformations.

Understanding Stomach Ulcers

Stomach ulcers, also known as gastric ulcers or peptic ulcers, are a common yet often misunderstood medical condition. These painful sores that develop on the inner lining of the stomach or the upper part of the small intestine can significantly impact a person's quality of life. To comprehend stomach ulcers fully, it's essential to explore their causes, symptoms, risk factors, and treatment options.

Causes of Stomach Ulcers

Helicobacter pylori (H. pylori) Infection: The most common cause of stomach ulcers is infection with the bacterium Helicobacter pylori. H. pylori can weaken the protective mucous lining of the stomach and duodenum, making them more susceptible to damage from stomach acid.

Nonsteroidal Anti-Inflammatory Drugs (NSAIDs): Regular or prolonged use of NSAIDs, such as aspirin, ibuprofen, or naproxen, can irritate the stomach lining, disrupt the mucous barrier, and contribute to the development of ulcers.

Excessive Stomach Acid: Overproduction of stomach acid, a condition known as hyperacidity, can overwhelm the stomach's natural defenses, leading to ulcer formation

Stress and Lifestyle Factors: While stress itself doesn't directly cause ulcers; it can exacerbate the condition. Smoking and excessive alcohol consumption can also increase the risk of developing ulcers.

Common Symptoms

Burning Pain: The hallmark symptom of stomach ulcers is a burning or gnawing pain in the upper abdomen, often between meals or during the night.

Nausea and Vomiting: Some individuals may experience nausea, vomiting, or bloating.

Loss of Appetite: Ulcers can lead to a decreased appetite and unintended weight loss.

Bleeding: In severe cases, ulcers can cause internal bleeding, which may result in dark, tarry stools or vomiting blood.

Indigestion: Frequent indigestion or heartburn can be indicative of an underlying ulcer.

Risk Factors

Several factors can increase the likelihood of developing stomach ulcers:

H. pylori Infection: Exposure to this bacterium, often through contaminated food or water, is a significant risk factor.

NSAID Use: Taking NSAIDs regularly, especially at high doses, can irritate the stomach lining.

Age: Stomach ulcers are more common in older adults.

Family History: A family history of ulcers can increase susceptibility.

Smoking and Alcohol: These lifestyle choices can weaken the stomach's natural defenses.

Alcohol Consumption: Excessive alcohol consumption can irritate the stomach lining and increase susceptibility to ulcers.

Stress: While stress itself doesn't directly cause ulcers, it can exacerbate existing ulcers and delay healing.

Chronic Medical Conditions: Certain medical conditions, such as liver disease, chronic obstructive pulmonary disease (COPD), and kidney failure, can elevate the risk of stomach ulcers.

Zollinger-Ellison Syndrome: This rare genetic condition leads to excessive production of stomach acid and significantly increases the risk of ulcers.

Dietary Factors: While dietary factors alone are not direct causes, a diet high in spicy foods or very acidic foods can aggravate existing ulcers.

Previous Ulcers: A history of previous ulcers increases the risk of recurrence.

Understanding both the causes and risk factors associated with stomach ulcers is crucial for early detection and effective prevention. Timely medical intervention, lifestyle modifications (such as quitting smoking and moderating alcohol intake), and managing underlying conditions can significantly reduce the risk and impact of stomach ulcers. If you suspect you have a stomach ulcer or are experiencing persistent symptoms, consult a healthcare professional for proper diagnosis and guidance on appropriate treatment and prevention measures.

Treatment Options

Treatment for stomach ulcers typically involves a combination of approaches:

Antibiotics: If an H. pylori infection is present, a course of antibiotics is prescribed to eradicate the bacterium.

Medications: Proton pump inhibitors (PPIs) and histamine receptor blockers (H2 blockers) are commonly used to reduce stomach acid production, allowing the ulcer to heal.

Lifestyle Changes: Avoiding trigger foods, quitting smoking, limiting alcohol intake, and managing stress can help prevent ulcer recurrence.

Follow-Up Care: Regular check-ups with a healthcare provider are essential to monitor healing and ensure that the treatment plan is effective.

Understanding stomach ulcers is the first step toward effective management and prevention. With proper medical care, lifestyle adjustments, and awareness of risk factors, individuals can overcome the challenges posed by stomach ulcers and lead healthier, more comfortable lives. If you suspect you have a stomach ulcer or are experiencing persistent symptoms, it is crucial to consult with a healthcare professional for a proper diagnosis and treatment.

Complications of Stomach Ulcers

If left untreated, stomach ulcers can lead to serious complications, including:

Bleeding Ulcers: Ulcers can cause internal bleeding, leading to anemia and potentially life-threatening conditions.

Perforation: In rare cases, ulcers can create a hole in the stomach or duodenum wall, causing a medical emergency.

Obstruction: Scarring from healing ulcers may narrow the digestive tract, obstructing the passage of food.

Understanding what stomach ulcers are and recognizing their symptoms is crucial for prompt diagnosis and appropriate treatment. Fortunately, most stomach ulcers can be effectively managed with medication, lifestyle changes, and, in some cases, antibiotics to treat an underlying H. pylori infection. If you suspect you have a stomach ulcer or are experiencing persistent symptoms, it is essential to consult a healthcare professional for a proper diagnosis and treatment plan.

Managing Ulcer Symptoms with Diet

Stomach ulcers, also known as gastric or peptic ulcers, can be painful and disruptive to daily life. While medical treatment is essential, adopting a stomach ulcer-friendly diet can significantly help manage symptoms and support the healing process. Here's how you can manage ulcer symptoms with a well-balanced diet:

1. Eat Foods That Promote Healing:

High-Fiber Foods: Include plenty of fruits, vegetables, and whole grains in your diet. These foods can help repair and protect the stomach lining.

Probiotics: Foods like yogurt, kefir, and fermented vegetables contain probiotics that promote a healthy gut, potentially aiding ulcer healing.

Lean Proteins: Choose lean protein sources such as tofu, fish, and poultry. Tissue healing is aided by protein.

2. Avoid Trigger Foods:

Spicy Foods: Highly spiced dishes can irritate the stomach lining, so it's best to avoid them.

Acidic Foods: Citrus fruits, tomatoes, and their derivatives (like orange juice and tomato sauce) can increase stomach acid production.

Caffeine: Coffee, tea, and caffeinated beverages can stimulate acid secretion and worsen ulcer symptoms.

Alcohol: Excessive alcohol consumption can irritate the stomach lining and hinder the healing process.

Fatty and Fried Foods: High-fat foods can increase stomach acid production and delay healing.

3. Opt for Smaller, Frequent Meals:

Instead of three large meals a day, consider eating smaller, more frequent meals. This approach can help reduce the production of stomach acid and prevent overloading the stomach.

4. Choose Soothing Liquids:

Herbal Teas: Chamomile, ginger, and licorice root teas can have soothing effects on the stomach.

Water: Maintaining adequate hydration is crucial. Water facilitates digestion by reducing stomach acid.

5. Be Mindful of Medications:

If you're prescribed medications like proton pump inhibitors (PPIs) or H2 blockers to reduce stomach acid, take them as directed by your healthcare provider.

6. Maintain a Food Diary:

Keeping a record of what you eat and how it affects your symptoms can help identify trigger foods and patterns that exacerbate discomfort.

7. Stay Elevated After Meals:

To prevent stomach acid from flowing back into the esophagus (acid reflux), consider staying upright for at least 2-3 hours after eating.

8. Stress Management:

Chronic stress can worsen ulcer symptoms. Incorporate stress-reduction techniques such as meditation, deep breathing, and exercise into your daily routine.

9. Avoid Smoking:

Smoking can slow the healing process of stomach ulcers and increase the risk of complications. Quitting smoking is highly recommended.

10. Consult a Dietitian:

For personalized dietary guidance, consider consulting a registered dietitian or nutritionist who specializes in gastrointestinal health. They can create a tailored meal plan to suit your specific needs.

Remember that while a stomach ulcer-friendly diet can help manage symptoms and support healing, it should be combined with medical treatment prescribed by your healthcare provider.

Chapter 1

Building a Stomach-Friendly Plate

For individuals dealing with stomach ulcers or other digestive issues, constructing a stomach-friendly plate is essential to minimize discomfort, support healing, and promote overall well-being. By choosing the right foods and adopting mindful eating habits, you can create meals that are gentle on your stomach.

Here's how to build a stomach-friendly plate:

1. Start with a Lean Protein Source:

Incorporate lean protein options like skinless poultry, fish, tofu, or legumes. These proteins are less likely to irritate your stomach compared to fatty or heavily processed meats.

2. Add Fiber-Rich Foods:

Include fruits, vegetables, and whole grains. Fiber promotes intestinal health and facilitates digestion. Opt for easily digestible options like bananas, cooked carrots, or brown rice.

3. Choose Good Fats:

Opt for healthy fats such as avocados, olive oil, and nuts in moderation. These facts are less likely to trigger excessive stomach acid production.

4. Avoid Spicy and Acidic Foods:

Steer clear of spicy dishes and acidic foods like citrus fruits, tomatoes, and vinegar-based dressings, as they can aggravate stomach ulcers.

5. Mind Your Portions:

Limit the quantity of food you eat in order to avoid filling up your stomach with too many calories, which may bring about discomfort.

6. Incorporate Probiotics:

Consider adding yogurt or kefir with live cultures to your meal plan. These probiotic-rich foods can support a healthy gut microbiome.

7. Sip Fluids:

Drink fluids throughout the day, but avoid large quantities during meals, as excessive liquid can dilute stomach acid needed for digestion. Sip water or soothing herbal teas between meals.

8. Be Mindful of Seasonings:

Use mild seasonings like ginger, basil, or turmeric instead of strong spices to flavor your food. These spices are less likely to irritate the stomach.

9. Avoid Trigger Beverages:

Stay away from alcohol, carbonated drinks, and caffeinated beverages, as they can increase stomach acid production.

10. Eat Slowly and Chew Thoroughly:

Chew your meal well, taking your time to enjoy every bite. This facilitates digestion and lessens the possibility of swallowing air, which can cause pain and bloating.

11. Stay Upright After Meals:

Try to remain upright for at least 2-3 hours after eating to prevent acid reflux or heartburn.

12. Keep a Food Diary:

Maintain a journal of what you eat and how it affects your symptoms. This can help identify trigger foods and patterns that worsen discomfort.

13. Consult a Healthcare Professional:

If you're unsure about which foods to include or avoid, or if your symptoms persist or worsen, consult a healthcare provider or a registered dietitian with expertise in gastrointestinal health.

Remember that building a stomach-friendly plate may involve some trial and error to identify foods and eating habits that work best for you. It's essential to work closely with your healthcare team to develop a personalized meal plan that addresses your specific needs and supports the healing process. With patience and diligence, you can create meals that are both gentle on your stomach and nourishing for your body.

The Basics of a Stomach Ulcer Diet

A stomach ulcer diet plays a crucial role in managing the symptoms of peptic ulcers, promoting healing, and reducing the risk of complications. The primary goal of this diet is to minimize stomach irritation, control stomach acid production, and provide the necessary nutrients for the healing process.

Here are the basics of a stomach ulcer diet:

1. Choose Lean Proteins:

Lean protein options include fish, tofu, skinless chicken, and lentils. These proteins are easier to digest and less likely to trigger excess stomach acid production compared to fatty meats.

2. Embrace High-Fiber Foods:

Eat a diet rich in fruits, vegetables, and whole grains. Fiber aids in digestion and helps maintain regular bowel movements. However, select fruits and vegetables that are not too acidic and choose whole grains like brown rice, oats, and whole wheat bread.

3. Good Fats, Not Bad Fats:

Prioritize healthy fats such as avocados, olive oil, and nuts in moderation. These fats can support overall health and are less likely to irritate the stomach.

4. Avoid Spicy and Acidic Foods:

Stay away from spicy dishes, citrus fruits, tomatoes, and vinegar-based dressings, as they can aggravate stomach ulcers and lead to discomfort.

5. Be Mindful of Seasonings:

Use mild seasonings like ginger, basil, and turmeric to flavor your food. These spices are less likely to irritate the stomach lining.

6. Limit or Avoid Trigger Beverages:

Restrict or eliminate alcohol, carbonated drinks, and caffeinated beverages like coffee and tea, as they can stimulate stomach acid production and worsen ulcer symptoms.

7. Eat Smaller, Frequent Meals:

Aim for five or six smaller meals throughout the day, rather than three large ones. This approach can help reduce stomach irritation and prevent overloading the digestive system.

8. Include Probiotics:

Incorporate probiotic-rich foods like yogurt or kefir with live cultures. Probiotics can help maintain a healthy gut microbiome and support digestion.

9. Sip Fluids Between Meals:

Drink fluids throughout the day, but avoid consuming large quantities during meals, as excessive liquid can dilute stomach acid needed for digestion. Instead, sip water or soothing herbal teas between meals.

10. Eat Mindfully:

Practice mindful eating by chewing your food thoroughly, savoring each bite, and eating in a relaxed environment. This can aid digestion and reduce the risk of swallowing excess air, which can lead to bloating.

11. Maintain an Upright Position:

Try to remain upright for at least 2-3 hours after eating to prevent acid reflux or heartburn.

12. Keep a Food Diary:

Note your food intake and how it impacts your symptoms. This can help identify trigger foods and patterns that worsen discomfort.

13. Consult a Healthcare Professional:

For personalized dietary guidance and to ensure you're meeting your nutritional needs, consult a healthcare provider or a registered dietitian with expertise in gastrointestinal health.

Adhering to a stomach ulcer diet is essential for symptom management and ulcer healing. However, it's crucial to work closely with your healthcare team to tailor the diet to your specific needs and monitor your progress. With patience and dedication to a stomach-friendly eating plan, you can alleviate discomfort and support the healing process for a healthier digestive system.

Balancing Nutrients

Balancing nutrients is a fundamental aspect of maintaining optimal health and well-being. Proper nutrient balance ensures that our bodies receive the essential vitamins, minerals, and macronutrients (carbohydrates, proteins, and fats) needed for growth, energy, and overall functioning. Achieving this balance is crucial for preventing deficiencies, supporting bodily processes, and reducing the risk of chronic diseases.

Here's why balancing nutrients is essential and how to achieve it:

1. Macronutrients:

Carbohydrates: Carbohydrates provide the body's primary source of energy. Balancing carbohydrate intake is essential to maintain stable blood sugar levels and prevent energy spikes and crashes. Focus on complex carbohydrates like whole grains, fruits, and vegetables, while moderating refined sugars and processed foods.

Proteins: Proteins are crucial for building and repairing tissues. Balancing protein intake ensures that your body gets an adequate supply of essential amino acids. Include lean sources of protein like poultry, fish, legumes, and tofu in your diet.

Fats: Fats play a role in various bodily functions, including nutrient absorption and hormone production. Balancing fats involves prioritizing healthy unsaturated fats (found in nuts, seeds, avocados, and olive oil) while minimizing saturated and trans fats found in fried and processed foods.

2. Micronutrients:

Vitamins: Balancing vitamins is essential for overall health. Eating a diverse range of foods, including fruits, vegetables, whole grains, and lean proteins, can help ensure that you get a wide array of vitamins, including A, C, D, E, and K.

Minerals: Minerals like calcium, magnesium, potassium, and iron are vital for various bodily functions, including bone health, muscle function, and oxygen transport. Balancing minerals can be achieved by consuming a variety of nutrient-rich foods and, if necessary, taking supplements under the guidance of a healthcare provider.

3. Fiber:

Balancing dietary fiber is essential for digestive health and regulating blood sugar levels. Fiber-rich foods like whole grains, fruits, vegetables, and legumes help maintain proper bowel function and can lower the risk of certain chronic diseases.

4. Hydration:

Balancing fluid intake is crucial for overall well-being. Digestion, circulation, and temperature control all require water. Listen to your body's thirst cues, and aim to drink enough water throughout the day to stay properly hydrated.

5. Antioxidants:

Balancing antioxidants is vital for protecting cells from damage caused by free radicals. Antioxidant-rich foods like berries, leafy greens, and nuts can help neutralize harmful compounds in the body.

6. Individualized Nutrition:

Nutrient needs can vary widely among individuals based on factors like age, gender, activity level, and underlying health conditions. It's essential to consider your unique nutritional requirements and consult a healthcare provider or registered dietitian for personalized guidance.

7. Moderation and Variety:

Balancing nutrients is not about strict diets but rather about moderation and variety. Including a wide range of foods in your diet ensures that you receive the full spectrum of essential nutrients.

8. Mindful Eating:

Paying attention to hunger and fullness cues, practicing portion control, and enjoying meals without distractions can help you maintain a balanced approach to nutrition.

Balancing nutrients is a dynamic process that requires ongoing attention to your dietary choices and nutritional needs. By prioritizing a diverse, whole-food-based diet and consulting with healthcare professionals when necessary, you can achieve and maintain optimal nutrient balance for long-term health and vitality.

Portion Control

Portion control is a fundamental aspect of maintaining a healthy diet and achieving or maintaining a healthy weight. It involves being mindful of the amount of food you consume at each meal or snack, which is critical for managing calorie intake, preventing overeating, and promoting overall well-being. Here's why portion control matters and how to practice it effectively:

Why Portion Control Matters:

Calorie Management: You may control your calorie consumption by practicing portion management. Consuming more calories than your body needs can lead to weight gain, while consistently consuming fewer calories can lead to weight loss.

Prevents Overeating: It helps prevent overeating, a common contributor to obesity and digestive discomfort. Eating excessively can strain the digestive system and lead to feelings of lethargy and discomfort.

Balanced Nutrition: Portion control ensures a balanced intake of nutrients. It allows you to allocate space on your plate for different food groups, including vegetables, lean proteins, whole grains, and healthy fats, promoting a well-rounded diet.

Mindful Eating: Practicing portion control encourages mindful eating, which means paying attention to hunger and fullness cues, savoring each bite, and eating without distractions. This enhances your relationship with food and improves satisfaction.

How to Practice Portion Control:

Use Smaller Plates and Bowls: Choosing smaller dishes can visually trick your brain into thinking you have a larger portion of food, promoting satisfaction with smaller servings.

Measure Portions: Invest in a set of measuring cups and a kitchen scale to accurately measure food portions. This is especially helpful when preparing meals at home.

Learn Visual Cues: Acquaint oneself with visual signals to make accurate portion estimation. For example, a serving of meat should be about the size of a deck of cards, a cup of cooked pasta is approximately the size of a tennis ball, and a teaspoon of oil is roughly the size of a poker chip.

Split Restaurant Meals: When dining out, consider sharing an entree with a friend or asking for a to-go box to portion out half of your meal before you start eating.

Use Your Hand as a Guide: Your hand can serve as a convenient portion control tool. For example, a fist can represent a serving of vegetables, and the palm of your hand can approximate a serving of protein.

Avoid Eating Directly from Packages: Eating directly from a bag or container makes it easy to lose track of how much you've consumed. Instead, portion snacks into a small bowl.

Practice Mindful Eating: Eat mindfully—savor every bite, eat slowly, and pay attention to your body's signals of hunger and fullness. Put down your utensils between bites to pace yourself.

Plan Meals and Snacks: Plan meals and snacks in advance, and portion out servings to avoid spontaneous and often oversized eating.

Listen to Your Body: Eat when you're hungry and stop when you're satisfied. Steer clear of eating out of habit, stress, or boredom.

Stay Hydrated: Sometimes, thirst can be mistaken for hunger. Drinking water before a meal can help control portion sizes by ensuring you're not confusing thirst with hunger.

Practicing portion control is a sustainable approach to achieving and maintaining a healthy weight while enjoying a balanced and satisfying diet. It allows you to savor your food, nourish your body, and maintain a positive relationship with eating. By paying attention to portion sizes, you can make informed choices that support your health and well-being.

Meal Frequency

Meal frequency, or the number of times you eat in a day, is a crucial aspect of your overall eating pattern and can significantly impact your health, metabolism, and energy levels. Finding the right balance in meal frequency is essential for individual well-being and can vary based on personal preferences, lifestyle, and specific health goals. Here's a closer look at meal frequency and its implications for health:

Key Factors to Consider:

Energy Balance: One of the primary factors influencing meal frequency is energy balance. The number of calories you consume throughout the day should align with your energy expenditure to maintain or achieve a healthy weight.

Hunger and Appetite: Pay attention to your body's hunger and appetite cues. Eating when you're genuinely hungry and stopping when you're satisfied can help regulate meal frequency.

Nutrient Timing: The timing of your meals can affect how your body processes nutrients. Some people benefit from evenly spaced meals, while others may prefer intermittent fasting or fewer, larger meals.

Lifestyle and Schedule: Your daily routine and commitments can influence meal frequency. People with busy schedules may opt for smaller, more frequent meals, while those with flexible schedules may prefer larger, less frequent meals.

Metabolism: Meal frequency can influence metabolic rate, but the impact varies among individuals. Some studies suggest that eating smaller, frequent meals may slightly increase metabolism, while others show no significant difference compared to fewer, larger meals.

Meal Frequency Options:

Three Square Meals: Traditional meal patterns involve three main meals per day: breakfast, lunch, and dinner. This approach works well for many people and aligns with societal norms.

Snacking: Incorporating snacks between meals can help curb hunger and provide sustained energy. However, it's important to choose nutritious snacks rather than highly processed, calorie-dense options.

Intermittent Fasting: This strategy alternates between eating and fasting intervals. The 16/8 method, which involves fasting for 16 hours and eating within an 8-hour window, and the 5:2 strategy, which involves eating regularly for five days then substantially cutting calories for two non-consecutive days, are two popular approaches.

Multiple Small Meals: Eating five or six smaller meals throughout the day can help control appetite and blood sugar levels, particularly for individuals with diabetes.

Considerations for Health and Well-Being:
Nutrient Intake: Regardless of meal frequency, prioritize a balanced diet rich in fruits, vegetables, lean proteins, whole grains, and healthy fats. Adequate nutrient intake is more important than meal timing.

Portion Control: Regardless of meal frequency, practice portion control to avoid overeating. Measuring serving sizes and being mindful of hunger and fullness cues can help maintain calorie balance.

Individual Variation: Recognize that what works for one person may not work for another. Experiment with meal frequency to find the eating pattern that best suits your body, lifestyle, and health goals.

Hydration: Stay well-hydrated throughout the day, regardless of your meal frequency. It is vital for general health to drink water.

Consult a Healthcare Professional: If you have specific health conditions or dietary concerns, consider seeking guidance from a healthcare provider or registered dietitian who can provide personalized recommendations.

In conclusion, there is no one-size-fits-all approach to meal frequency. Finding the right balance that suits your individual needs, preferences, and lifestyle is key to maintaining a healthy and sustainable eating pattern. Focus on nutrient quality, portion control, and mindful eating, and consult with a healthcare professional if you have specific dietary goals or concerns.

Foods to Include

A balanced diet is essential for maintaining good health, providing the body with the necessary nutrients, energy, and support for various bodily functions. Including a wide variety of foods in your diet ensures you get a full spectrum of essential nutrients. Here are some key foods to include for a balanced and nourishing diet:

1. Fruits and Vegetables:

Leafy Greens: Spinach, kale, Swiss chard, and collard greens are rich in vitamins, minerals, and antioxidants.

Colorful Fruits: Berries, citrus fruits, apples, and bananas provide essential vitamins, fiber, and antioxidants.

Cruciferous Vegetables: Broccoli, cauliflower, Brussels sprouts, and cabbage are packed with nutrients and cancer-fighting compounds.

Root Vegetables: Carrots, sweet potatoes, and beets are high in fiber, vitamins, and minerals.

2. Whole Grains:

Brown Rice: A healthy source of complex carbohydrates, fiber, and essential nutrients.

Quinoa: A complete protein source containing all essential amino acids, as well as vitamins and minerals.

Oats: Rich in soluble fiber, which supports heart health, and provides sustained energy.

Whole Wheat: Whole wheat bread, pasta, and cereals offer fiber and nutrients compared to refined grains.

3. Lean Proteins:

Poultry: Turkey and skinless chicken are great sources of lean protein.

Fish: Fatty fish like salmon, mackerel, and trout provide omega-3 fatty acids, which support heart and brain health.

Legumes: Chickpeas, lentils, and beans are rich in fibre, protein, and other minerals.

Tofu and Tempeh: Plant-based protein sources that are rich in nutrients and suitable for vegetarians and vegans.

4. Healthy Fats:

Avocado: A source of heart-healthy monounsaturated fats, fiber, and various vitamins and minerals.

Nuts and Seeds: Healthy fats, protein, and important elements are offered by almonds, walnuts, chia seeds, and flaxseeds.

Olive Oil: Extra virgin olive oil is a staple of the Mediterranean diet and is rich in monounsaturated fats and antioxidants.

5. Dairy or Dairy Alternatives:

Greek Yogurt: High in protein and probiotics, which support gut health.

Milk Alternatives: Soy milk, almond milk, and oat milk provide calcium and are suitable for those with lactose intolerance or dairy allergies.

6. Proteins:

Eggs: A rich source of protein, vitamins, and minerals. Eggs can be prepared in various ways and are a versatile ingredient.

Lean Meats: Lean cuts of beef or pork provide high-quality protein and essential nutrients.

7. Hydration:

Water: Staying well-hydrated is essential for overall health. Water aids in temperature regulation, circulation, and digestion.

8. Herbs and Spices:

Turmeric: Known for its anti-inflammatory properties.

Garlic: Adds flavor and has potential health benefits.

Cinnamon: May help regulate blood sugar levels.

9. Variety:

Include a wide variety of foods in your diet to ensure you get a broad spectrum of nutrients. Rotate your choices to prevent dietary monotony.

10. Portion Control:

Pay attention to portion sizes to avoid overeating, even when consuming healthy foods.

Remember that a balanced diet is about overall eating patterns rather than individual foods. Strive for moderation, mindful eating, and a diverse range of nutrient-rich foods to support your health and well-being.

Lean Proteins

Lean proteins are a fundamental element of a healthy diet, offering essential nutrients and supporting various bodily functions. These protein sources are characterized by their lower fat content compared to fattier cuts of meat, making them a preferred choice for those aiming to maintain or achieve a healthy weight and reduce saturated fat intake.

Here's why lean proteins are important and some excellent sources to include in your diet:

Importance of Lean Proteins:

Muscle Maintenance and Growth: Proteins are essential for the repair and growth of muscles, making them vital for maintaining a healthy body composition.

Satiety and Weight Management: Protein-rich foods are more filling and can help control appetite, making them an excellent choice for those looking to manage their weight.

Nutrient Density: Lean proteins provide essential nutrients like vitamins (e.g., B vitamins) and minerals (e.g., iron, zinc) without excessive calories from fat.

Heart Health: Choosing lean proteins can help reduce saturated fat intake, which is associated with a lower risk of heart disease.

Blood Sugar Regulation: Protein can help stabilize blood sugar levels, which is especially beneficial for individuals with diabetes or those at risk of developing the condition.

Excellent Sources of Lean Proteins:

Poultry: Skinless chicken and turkey breast are lean choices that are versatile and high in protein. Avoid frying and choose healthier cooking methods like grilling, roasting, or baking.

Fish: Fatty fish like salmon, mackerel, sardines, and trout are rich in heart-healthy omega-3 fatty acids. White fish like cod and tilapia are also lean options.

Seafood: Shrimp, crab, and scallops are low in fat and provide protein, vitamins, and minerals. Opt for grilled or poached seafood dishes.

Lean Cuts of Meat: Choose lean cuts of beef, pork, or lamb, such as sirloin, tenderloin, or loin chops. Trim visible fat before cooking and use cooking methods that require minimal added fats.

Legumes: Beans, lentils, and chickpeas are plant-based sources of protein that are low in fat and high in fiber. Vegetarians and vegans can also eat them.

Tofu and Tempeh: These soy-based products are rich in protein and are versatile ingredients in vegetarian and vegan diets.

Low-Fat Dairy: Greek yogurt, low-fat or fat-free milk, and cottage cheese are dairy sources of lean protein. They also provide calcium and other nutrients.

Eggs: Eggs are a high-quality source of protein, and the egg white is particularly lean. Enjoy eggs as a versatile ingredient in various dishes.

Lean Deli Meats: When choosing deli meats, opt for lean options like turkey or chicken breast. Seek for goods with reduced salt levels.

Plant-Based Proteins: Beyond meat alternatives, there are many plant-based proteins sources like seitan, edamame, and various meat substitutes made from beans and vegetables.

When incorporating lean proteins into your diet, it's important to practice healthy cooking methods like grilling, baking, steaming, or poaching to keep added fats to a minimum.

Additionally, combine lean proteins with a variety of vegetables, whole grains, and healthy fats to create balanced and nutritious meals. This approach ensures you receive a wide range of essential nutrients and supports your overall health and well-being.

High-Fiber Choices

Dietary fiber is a crucial component of a healthy diet, known for its numerous health benefits, including supporting digestive health, regulating blood sugar levels, and aiding weight management. High-fiber choices are foods that are rich in dietary fiber, and incorporating them into your diet can promote overall well-being.

Here's why dietary fiber is important and a selection of high-fiber foods to consider:

The Importance of Dietary Fiber:

Digestive Health: Dietary fibre encourages regular bowel movements and helps avoid constipation by giving the stool more volume. It also supports a healthy gut microbiome, which is essential for overall digestion.

Blood Sugar Control: High-fiber foods can slow the absorption of sugar, helping to stabilize blood sugar levels. For those who already have diabetes or are at risk of getting it, this is especially crucial.

Weight Management: Fiber-rich foods are typically filling and can help control appetite, making it easier to manage portion sizes and overall calorie intake.

Heart Health: A diet high in fiber can lower cholesterol levels and reduce the risk of heart disease. Specifically, soluble fibre binds to cholesterol and draws it out of the body.

Colorectal Health: Consuming a diet rich in fiber may lower the risk of developing colorectal cancer.

High-Fiber Choices:

Whole Grains:

Oats: Oatmeal and oat bran are rich sources of soluble fiber, which can help lower cholesterol levels.

Quinoa: A complete protein source with both soluble and insoluble fiber.

Whole Wheat: Opt for whole wheat bread, pasta, and cereals to increase fiber intake.

Legumes:

Beans: Black beans, kidney beans, chickpeas, and lentils are all high in fiber and can be added to soups, salads, and stews.

Fruits:

Berries: Blueberries, strawberries, raspberries, and blackberries are particularly high in fiber and antioxidants.

Apples: An apple with its skin provides a good amount of fiber and makes for a convenient snack.

Pears: Like apples, pears are high in fiber and make for a delicious and nutritious addition to your diet.

Vegetables:

Broccoli: Rich in fiber, vitamins, and minerals, broccoli is a versatile and nutritious vegetable.

Carrots: Carrots are not only crunchy but also high in fiber and vitamins.

Spinach: Dark leafy greens like spinach offer fiber and a range of other nutrients.

Nuts and Seeds:

Almonds: Almonds are high in fiber and healthy fats, making them a satisfying and nutritious snack.

Chia Seeds: Chia seeds are a superfood packed with fiber and omega-3 fatty acids.

Bran: Wheat bran, oat bran, and rice bran can be added to cereals, yogurt, or smoothies to increase fiber content.

Psyllium Husk: Psyllium husk is a soluble fiber supplement that can be mixed with water or added to foods like oatmeal to boost fiber intake.

Popcorn: Air-popped popcorn is a whole grain snack that provides fiber while being relatively low in calories.

Vegetable Skins: When you consume vegetables like potatoes, sweet potatoes, and zucchini, leave the skin on for added fiber.

Fruit with Skin: Whenever possible, eat fruits like grapes, kiwi, and peaches with the skin, as it contains additional fiber.

When incorporating high-fiber choices into your diet, it's important to increase your fiber intake gradually and drink plenty of water to prevent digestive discomfort. Aim to diversify your fiber sources to receive a wide range of nutrients and health benefits. A balanced diet that includes high-fiber foods can contribute to improved overall health and well-being.

Probiotic-Rich Options

When taken in sufficient quantities, living bacteria known as probiotics can provide a number of health advantages. Because they support the maintenance of a balanced population of microorganisms in the gut, these bacteria are frequently referred to as "good" or "friendly" bacteria. Probiotic-rich foods and supplements can support digestive health, boost the immune system, and even contribute to overall well-being. Here's a look at the importance of probiotics and some excellent sources to consider:

The Importance of Probiotics:

Gut Health: Probiotics play a vital role in maintaining a balanced gut microbiome. A diverse and healthy gut microbiome is associated with improved digestion, nutrient absorption, and overall well-being.

Immune Support: A significant portion of the immune system resides in the gut. Probiotics can help support the immune system by promoting a favorable environment for immune cells to function.

Digestive Comfort: Probiotics may alleviate digestive discomfort and help manage conditions like irritable bowel syndrome (IBS) and diarrhea.

Mental Health: There may be a connection between gut health and mental wellness, according to recent studies. Probiotics may play a role in mood regulation and mental health.

Probiotic-Rich Options:

Yogurt: One of the most well-known foods high in probiotics is yoghurt. A label that reads "live and active cultures" should be your first clue. Greek yogurt, kefir, and skier are especially rich in probiotics.

Fermented Foods:

Sauerkraut: Fermented cabbage that is high in probiotics and vitamins.

Kimchi: A spicy fermented Korean side dish made from vegetables, primarily cabbage and radishes.

Kombucha: A fermented tea beverage that contains live probiotic cultures.

Miso: A traditional Japanese seasoning made by fermenting soybeans with salt and koji fungus.

Tempeh: A fermented soybean product that is rich in probiotics and protein.

Pickles (Brine-Cured): Pickles that are made using fermentation and not just vinegar may contain probiotics.

Buttermilk: Similar to yogurt, buttermilk contains live cultures and can be used in cooking and baking.

Soft Cheeses: Certain soft cheeses like gouda and cottage cheese can contain probiotics, but the content may vary.

Non-Dairy Alternatives: Some non-dairy options like coconut milk yogurt and almond milk yogurt are fortified with probiotics.

Supplements: Probiotic supplements are available in various forms, including capsules, tablets, powders, and gummies. Before using supplements, it is best to speak with a healthcare provider, particularly if you have any particular health issues.

Prebiotic-Rich Foods: Prebiotics are non-digestible fibers that feed beneficial gut bacteria. Foods like garlic, onions, leeks, and asparagus are prebiotic-rich and can complement probiotic intake.

Probiotic Fortified Foods: Some breakfast cereals, granola bars, and beverages may be fortified with probiotics. Check the product labels for details.

When incorporating probiotic-rich foods into your diet, aim for variety to maximize the diversity of beneficial microorganisms in your gut. Also, consider introducing probiotics gradually to allow your digestive system to adapt. If you have specific health concerns or conditions, consult with a healthcare professional or registered dietitian for personalized guidance on probiotic intake. By including probiotic-rich options in your diet, you can promote gut health and contribute to overall wellness.

Hydration and Herbal Teas

Proper hydration is essential for overall health and well-being. Water is the foundation of life and plays a crucial role in numerous bodily functions, including digestion, circulation, temperature regulation, and the elimination of waste products. While plain water is the primary source of hydration, herbal teas offer a delightful and flavorful way to stay hydrated while providing additional health benefits.

Here's a look at the importance of hydration and the benefits of herbal teas:

The Importance of Hydration:

Optimal Body Function: Water is a key component of cells, tissues, and organs, enabling them to perform their functions efficiently.

Digestive Health: Adequate hydration is vital for digestion. Water helps break down food and move it through the digestive tract, preventing constipation.

Temperature Regulation: Sweating is the body's natural cooling mechanism, and sufficient hydration helps regulate body temperature, especially in hot weather or during physical activity.

Nutrient Transport: Water facilitates the transport of nutrients from the digestive system to the cells where they are needed for energy and overall health.

Detoxification: Proper hydration supports the kidneys and liver in removing waste products and toxins from the body.

Herbal Teas for Hydration and Health:

Herbal teas, also known as tisanes, are caffeine-free infusions made from various plants, herbs, and spices. They are not only a flavorful way to stay hydrated but also offer numerous health benefits:

Mint Tea: Peppermint and spearmint teas are refreshing and may help soothe digestive discomfort, alleviate headaches, and relieve nausea.

Chamomile Tea: Chamomile tea has calming properties and is often used to promote relaxation, reduce anxiety, and support sleep.

Ginger Tea: Ginger tea is known for its anti-inflammatory and digestive benefits. It can help relieve nausea, indigestion, and menstrual discomfort.

Hibiscus Tea: Hibiscus tea is rich in antioxidants and may help lower blood pressure, support heart health, and boost the immune system.

Green Tea: While green tea contains caffeine, it is lower in caffeine compared to black tea and coffee. It is rich in antioxidants and has been associated with various health benefits, including improved brain function and reduced risk of chronic diseases.

Rooibos Tea: Rooibos, or red bush tea, is caffeine-free and high in antioxidants. It might strengthen the immune system and promote heart health.

Lemon Balm Tea: Lemon balm tea is calming and may help reduce stress and improve mood. It is also used to alleviate digestive discomfort.

Dandelion Tea: Dandelion tea is believed to support liver and kidney function, aid digestion, and act as a diuretic.

Cinnamon Tea: Cinnamon tea is warming and may help regulate blood sugar levels and lower inflammation.

Peppermint Tea: Peppermint tea is refreshing and can soothe digestive issues, reduce headaches, and relieve respiratory symptoms.

Tips for Hydration with Herbal Teas:

Enjoy herbal teas hot or iced, depending on your preference and the weather.

Limit or avoid adding sugar or honey to your herbal teas to keep them low in calories and sugar.

Experiment with combinations of herbs and spices to create unique flavor profiles.

Be mindful of individual sensitivities or allergies to specific herbs or ingredients.

Keep a variety of herbal teas on hand to cater to different moods and needs.

Incorporating herbal teas into your daily routine can enhance your hydration while providing a range of potential health benefits.

Remember that while herbal teas can contribute to hydration, they should not be the sole source of your daily water intake. Drinking plain water and herbal teas in combination is an excellent way to stay properly hydrated while enjoying a variety of flavors and potential health perks.

Foods to Avoid

Maintaining a healthy diet involves not only selecting the right foods but also being mindful of the foods to avoid. Certain foods and ingredients can contribute to health problems when consumed excessively or regularly. By identifying and limiting these items in your diet, you can work towards better health and well-being.

Here are some foods to consider avoiding or consuming in moderation:

1. Sugary Beverages:

Soda: Regular consumption of sugary soda has been linked to weight gain, obesity, type 2 diabetes, and dental problems.

Fruit Juice: Many fruit juices are high in added sugars and lack the fiber found in whole fruits. Opt for whole fruits or unsweetened fruit juice options.

Energy Drinks: These beverages often contain high levels of caffeine and sugar and can lead to energy crashes and increased heart rate.

2. Processed Snacks:

Chips: Potato chips, corn chips, and other snack chips are typically high in unhealthy fats, salt, and calories.

Candy: Candy is loaded with added sugars and provides little to no nutritional value.

Processed Snack Bars: Many granola bars and snack bars are packed with sugar, unhealthy fats, and artificial additives.

3. Sugary Cereals:

Some cereals marketed to children are loaded with sugar. Select wholegrain cereals with less added sugar.

4. Fast Food:

Foods that are fast food, such as burgers, fries, and fried chicken, are often heavy in calories, sodium, and bad fats. Limit their consumption.

5. Processed Meats:

Processed meats like bacon, sausages, hot dogs, and deli meats are often high in sodium and may contain preservatives linked to health risks like cancer.

6. Sugary Desserts:

Pastries, cakes, cookies, and ice cream are rich in added sugars and unhealthy fats. Enjoy these treats in moderation.

7. Sugary Breakfast Cereals:

Many breakfast cereals targeted at children are high in added sugars. Opt for whole-grain cereals with minimal added sugar.

8. Trans Fats:

Trans fats, often found in partially hydrogenated oils, are associated with heart disease. Check food labels for trans-fat content and avoid products that contain them.

9. High-Sodium Foods:

High-sodium foods like processed soups, canned goods, and certain restaurant dishes can contribute to high blood pressure and heart disease. Choose low-sodium alternatives when possible.

10. Sugary Coffee Drinks:

Many coffee shop beverages are loaded with added sugars and unhealthy fats. Consider ordering plain coffee or choosing lower-calorie options.

11. Alcohol:

Excessive alcohol consumption can have various negative health effects, including liver disease, addiction, and increased risk of accidents.

12. Artificial Sweeteners:

While some people use artificial sweeteners as a sugar substitute, their long-term health effects are still being studied. It's advisable to limit their use and opt for natural sweeteners like honey or maple syrup when needed.

13. High-Fat Dairy Products:

Full-fat dairy products can be high in saturated fats, which may raise LDL (bad) cholesterol levels. Consider lower-fat or plant-based alternatives.

14. Highly Processed Foods:

Foods with long ingredient lists containing artificial additives, colors, and preservatives should be consumed sparingly. Whenever possible, choose whole, minimally processed foods.

Remember that moderation is key when it comes to less healthy foods. Occasional indulgences are okay, but making them a regular part of your diet can have negative consequences for your health. Focus on a balanced diet that includes a variety of whole foods like fruits, vegetables, whole grains, lean proteins, and healthy fats to support your overall health and well-being.

Spicy and Acidic Foods

Spicy and acidic foods can add excitement and flavor to your meals, but they can also have various effects on your health and digestive system. While both types of foods offer unique tastes and culinary experiences, it's essential to be mindful of their potential impacts and consume them in moderation. Here's a closer look at spicy and acidic foods and some tips for incorporating them into your diet wisely:

Spicy Foods:

Spicy foods get their heat from compounds like capsaicin, found in chili peppers. While they can offer several health benefits, they can also have drawbacks:

Benefits:

Metabolism Boost: Capsaicin may help with weight management by momentarily speeding up metabolism.

Pain Relief: Topical capsaicin creams may help relieve pain, especially for conditions like arthritis.

Heart Health: Some research suggests that capsaicin may support heart health by reducing cholesterol levels and improving blood circulation.

Drawbacks:

Digestive Discomfort: Spicy foods can irritate the gastrointestinal tract, causing heartburn, acid reflux, or indigestion in some individuals.

Gastrointestinal Issues: Spicy foods can exacerbate conditions like irritable bowel syndrome (IBS) and may lead to diarrhea or abdominal pain.

Increased Body Temperature: Eating very spicy foods can lead to a temporary increase in body temperature and sweating, which may be uncomfortable in hot weather.

Tips for Consuming Spicy Foods:

Start Slow: If you're not accustomed to spicy foods, begin with milder options and gradually increase the level of spiciness as your tolerance grows.

Balance with Dairy: Dairy products like milk, yogurt, or cheese can help neutralize the heat from spicy foods.

Bland Accompaniments: Pair spicy dishes with mild sides like rice or bread to balance the flavors.

Stay Hydrated: Drink water to help alleviate the burning sensation, but avoid excessive consumption as it can spread the heat.

Be Mindful of Spices: Read labels and ask about the spiciness level when dining out to avoid unexpectedly spicy dishes.

Acidic Foods:

Acidic foods are those with a low pH level, typically containing high levels of acids like citric acid, malic acid, or acetic acid. These foods offer various culinary pleasures but also come with considerations:

Benefits:

Vitamin C: Many acidic foods are rich in vitamin C, which is essential for immune function, skin health, and wound healing.

Flavor Enhancement: Acids can enhance the flavors of dishes, making them more enjoyable.

Drawbacks:

Dental Health: Acidic foods and beverages can erode tooth enamel over time, leading to dental issues like cavities and sensitivity.

Digestive Discomfort: Acidic foods can trigger acid reflux or heartburn in some individuals.

Tips for Consuming Acidic Foods:

Moderation: Enjoy acidic foods in moderation to minimize potential dental and digestive issues.

Dental Care: Rinse your mouth with water after consuming acidic foods to help protect your teeth. Avoid brushing immediately after acidic foods, as it can further damage softened enamel.

Balanced Diet: Include a variety of foods in your diet to ensure you get a wide range of nutrients while minimizing the impact of acidic foods.

Antacid Medications: If you have chronic acid reflux or digestive issues, consult a healthcare professional who may recommend antacid medications or dietary changes.

Incorporating spicy and acidic foods into your diet can be a delightful experience, but it's important to be aware of their potential effects on your health and well-being. By consuming these foods in moderation, balancing them with other ingredients, and taking steps to mitigate their potential drawbacks, you can enjoy their flavors while maintaining good digestive health and overall wellness.

Caffeine and Carbonated Drinks

Caffeine and carbonated drinks are popular beverages enjoyed by people around the world. While they can provide a quick energy boost and a refreshing sensation, it's important to understand their impact on health and make informed choices when consuming them.

Here's a closer look at caffeine and carbonated drinks, their effects, and some considerations for responsible consumption:

Caffeine:

A natural stimulant, caffeine can be found in a variety of foods and drinks, such as tea, coffee, chocolate, and some soft drinks. It affects the central nervous system, increasing alertness and temporarily relieving fatigue. While caffeine offers potential benefits, such as improved cognitive function and enhanced exercise performance, it also has some drawbacks:

Benefits:

Alertness: Caffeine can help combat drowsiness and improve concentration, making it a popular choice for morning wake-ups or during work or study sessions.

Physical Performance: Caffeine can enhance physical endurance and reduce the perception of effort during exercise, making it a common ingredient in pre-workout supplements.

Antioxidants: Some caffeinated beverages, like green tea and black coffee, provide antioxidants that may have health benefits.

Drawbacks:

Insomnia: Usually in the afternoon or evening, caffeine consumption might disrupt sleep.

Anxiety and Jitters: High doses of caffeine can lead to feelings of restlessness, anxiety, and tremors.

Digestive Issues: Caffeine can stimulate gastric acid secretion, potentially leading to gastrointestinal discomfort in some individuals.

Dependency: Regular consumption can lead to caffeine dependency, with withdrawal symptoms like headaches and irritability when intake is reduced or stopped abruptly.

Heart Health: High caffeine intake may increase heart rate and blood pressure, which can be problematic for individuals with certain heart conditions.

Tips for Responsible Caffeine Consumption:

Moderation: Keep caffeine intake within recommended guidelines, which typically suggest up to 400 milligrams per day for most adults (about 4 cups of brewed coffee).

Timing: Avoid caffeine in the late afternoon or evening to minimize sleep disruption.

Hydration: Balance caffeinated beverages with plenty of water to stay adequately hydrated.

Individual Tolerance: Be mindful of your individual tolerance to caffeine, as some people are more sensitive to its effects.

Carbonated Drinks:

Carbonated drinks, often referred to as soda or soft drinks, are popular beverages that contain carbon dioxide gas, which creates effervescence and a characteristic fizzy sensation. These beverages come in a wide range of flavors and types, but many of them share certain health considerations:

Benefits:

Palate Pleasure: The effervescence and variety of flavors can make carbonated drinks enjoyable and refreshing.

Occasional Treat: As an occasional indulgence, carbonated drinks can be part of a balanced diet and provide a treat-like experience.

Drawbacks:

High Sugar Content: Many carbonated drinks are loaded with added sugars, which contribute to excess calorie intake and can lead to weight gain and related health issues.

Acidic Nature: Carbonated drinks can be acidic, potentially contributing to dental erosion and tooth decay.

Empty Calories: Sugary carbonated drinks provide little to no nutritional value, which can displace nutrient-dense foods in the diet.

Caffeine: Some carbonated drinks, like colas, contain caffeine, which can contribute to caffeine-related issues if consumed excessively.

Tips for Responsible Carbonated Drink Consumption:

Choose Wisely: Opt for sugar-free or low-sugar carbonated options to reduce sugar intake.

Moderation: Enjoy carbonated drinks as an occasional treat rather than a daily habit.

Oral Care: Rinse your mouth with water after consuming carbonated drinks to help protect tooth enamel.

Portion Control: Choose smaller serving sizes when available to manage calorie and sugar intake.

Consider Alternatives: Explore healthier beverage alternatives like sparkling water with a splash of fruit juice or herbal tea. Caffeine and carbonated drinks can be part of a balanced diet when consumed in moderation and with awareness of their potential effects on health. It's essential to make informed choices that align with your individual health goals and preferences while enjoying these beverages responsibly.

Alcohol and Smoking

Alcohol consumption and smoking are two common lifestyle choices that can have significant impacts on health. While moderate and responsible use of alcohol and avoiding smoking can have limited health risks, excessive or habitual consumption of alcohol and smoking tobacco are associated with a wide range of health problems. Here's a comprehensive look at the health risks and considerations associated with alcohol and smoking:

Alcohol:

Moderate Alcohol Consumption:

Moderate alcohol consumption, when done responsibly, is associated with some potential health benefits:

Heart Health: Some studies suggest that moderate alcohol consumption, particularly of red wine, may have cardiovascular benefits, including a potential reduction in the risk of heart disease.

Social Enjoyment: For many people, alcohol is a part of social and cultural gatherings and can contribute to relaxation and enjoyment in moderation.

Excessive Alcohol Consumption:

Excessive alcohol consumption, on the other hand, poses various health risks:

Addiction: Heavy drinking can lead to alcohol dependency, with physical and psychological withdrawal symptoms when consumption is reduced or stopped.

Liver Damage: Chronic alcohol abuse can cause liver damage, leading to conditions like fatty liver, alcoholic hepatitis, and cirrhosis.

Cancer Risk: Alcohol consumption is linked to an increased risk of several types of cancer, including mouth, throat, esophagus, liver, and breast cancer.

Mental Health: Alcohol misuse can contribute to mental health issues such as depression and anxiety.

Accidents and Injuries: Because alcohol affects judgement and coordination, there is a higher chance of mishaps and injury.

Responsible Alcohol Consumption:

If you decide to drink, you need make sure you do it sensibly:

Moderation: Stick to recommended guidelines, such as no more than one drink per day for women and up to two drinks per day for men.

Know Your Limit: Be aware of your own tolerance and never drink and drive.

Hydration: To stay hydrated in between alcoholic drinks, sip water.

Smoking:

Smoking tobacco is one of the leading causes of preventable death worldwide and is associated with numerous health risks:

Cancer: Smoking is the primary cause of lung cancer, and it's linked to cancers of the mouth, throat, esophagus, pancreas, bladder, and more.

Respiratory Issues: Smoking damages the respiratory system, leading to conditions like chronic obstructive pulmonary disease (COPD) and emphysema.

Heart Disease: Smoking increases the risk of heart disease, including heart attacks and stroke.

Addiction: Nicotine in tobacco is highly addictive, making it challenging to quit smoking.

Pregnancy Complications: Smoking during pregnancy can lead to complications like low birth weight and preterm birth.

Quitting Smoking:

Quitting smoking is one of the most beneficial decisions for your health:

Support: Seek support from healthcare professionals, smoking cessation programs, or support groups to increase your chances of quitting successfully.

Nicotine Replacement Therapy (NRT): Consider NRT options like nicotine gum, patches, or prescription medications to help manage withdrawal symptoms.

Lifestyle Changes: Adopt a healthier lifestyle with regular exercise and a balanced diet to support your efforts to quit.

Avoid Triggers: Identify and avoid situations or places that trigger the urge to smoke.

Patience: Be patient with yourself, as quitting smoking can be challenging, and it may take several attempts.

In summary, responsible alcohol consumption and avoiding smoking are essential for protecting your health. It's crucial to be aware of the health risks associated with these lifestyle choices and make informed decisions that prioritize your well-being. If you have concerns about your alcohol or smoking habits, consider seeking support and guidance from healthcare professionals or support groups to help you make positive changes for your health.

Chapter 2

Breakfasts to Soothe Your Stomach

When you wake up with a sensitive or upset stomach, it's essential to choose breakfast foods that are easy on your digestive system while providing necessary nutrients to start your day. Opting for soothing and gentle options can help alleviate discomfort and promote overall well-being.

Here are some breakfast ideas designed to soothe your stomach:

1. Oatmeal:

Oatmeal is a go-to breakfast choice for those with digestive discomfort. It's easy to digest, and its soluble fiber can help regulate bowel movements and ease indigestion.

Choose plain, unsweetened oatmeal and customize it with toppings like:

Sliced banana: Rich in potassium and easy to digest.

Applesauce: Gentle on the stomach and adds natural sweetness.

A sprinkle of ground flaxseeds: Provides additional fiber and healthy fats.

A drizzle of honey or a touch of cinnamon for flavor.

2. Yogurt:

Plain, low-fat yogurt contains probiotics, which can support a healthy gut. Probiotics are beneficial bacteria that promote digestion and may ease stomach discomfort. Avoid yogurt with added sugars, as they can exacerbate digestive issues.

Top your yogurt with:

Sliced, ripe bananas: Gentle on the stomach and a good source of potassium.

Fresh or frozen berries: Rich in antioxidants and fiber.

A dollop of honey for natural sweetness.

3. Rice Porridge (Congee):

Congee is a traditional Asian rice porridge known for its soothing properties. It's made by simmering rice in a generous amount of water until it reaches a creamy consistency.

Customize your congee with:

Shredded chicken or tofu: Provides protein while remaining gentle on the stomach.

Ginger: Known for its anti-nausea properties and pleasant flavor.

Scallions: Add a mild, onion-like flavor.

4. Scrambled Eggs:

Scrambled eggs are a protein-rich option that's usually well-tolerated. Be sure to cook them gently to avoid excessive oil or butter. You can add:

Mild, soft cheeses like ricotta or feta for extra creaminess.

Chopped spinach or cooked zucchini for added nutrients.

A slice of whole-grain toast or a small serving of rice for a balanced meal.

5. Herbal Teas:

Sipping on herbal teas can be soothing for an upset stomach. Peppermint, ginger, chamomile, and fennel teas are all known for their digestive benefits. Enjoy them plain or with a touch of honey.

6. Banana and Peanut Butter Sandwich:

A simple banana and peanut butter sandwich on whole-grain bread can provide a mix of carbohydrates, healthy fats, and protein. The banana is gentle on the stomach, while the peanut butter adds creaminess and flavor.

7. Mashed Avocado on Toast:

Avocados are a fantastic source of fibre and beneficial fats. Spread mashed avocado on whole-grain toast and season it with a pinch of salt and a dash of lemon or lime juice for added flavor.

8. Boiled or Poached Eggs with Toast:

Soft-boiled or poached eggs can be easier to digest than fried or hard-boiled eggs. To create a well-balanced supper, pair them with a slice of whole-grain toast.

When your stomach is feeling uneasy, it's essential to listen to your body and choose foods that will provide comfort and relief. These breakfast ideas are designed to be gentle on your stomach while delivering essential nutrients and soothing flavors to help you start your day on the right foot. Remember to stay hydrated with plain water or herbal teas throughout the morning to support your digestive system.

Oatmeal Delight

Oatmeal delight is a wholesome and customizable breakfast that combines the heartiness of oats with a wide range of flavorful toppings and additions. Whether you prefer a sweet, savory, or a balanced flavor profile, oatmeal provides the perfect canvas to create a satisfying and nutritious morning meal. Here's why oatmeal delight is a fantastic breakfast choice:

1. Nutritional Powerhouse:

Whole oats are the basis for muesli and are a great source of important nutrients.

Fiber: Oats are rich in soluble fiber, which can help regulate blood sugar levels, promote digestive health, and keep you feeling full.

Protein: Oats contain a decent amount of plant-based protein, making them a great breakfast option for vegetarians and vegans.

Vitamins and Minerals: Oats provide vitamins like B1 (thiamine) and B5 (pantothenic acid) and essential minerals such as manganese, phosphorus, and magnesium.

2. Heart Health:

Oats are well-known for their heart-healthy properties:

Reduced Cholesterol: The soluble fiber in oats, specifically beta-glucans, has been shown to lower LDL (bad) cholesterol levels, reducing the risk of heart disease.

Blood Pressure Control: Oats' magnesium content may help regulate blood pressure.

3. Sustained Energy:

The complex carbohydrates in oats provide a steady release of energy, helping you stay energized throughout the morning.

4. Customizable:

One of the best aspects of oatmeal delight is its versatility. You can tailor it to your taste preferences and dietary needs.

To get you going, consider these suggestions:

Sweet Toppings:

Fresh Berries: Add a burst of color and antioxidants with strawberries, blueberries, raspberries, or blackberries.

Bananas: Sliced bananas provide natural sweetness and creaminess.

Honey: Drizzle honey over your oatmeal for a natural sweetener.

Nuts: Add texture and healthy fats with almonds, walnuts, or pecans.

Nut Butter: A spoonful of almond, peanut, or cashew butter can create a creamy and satisfying oatmeal.

Savory Toppings:

Poached or Fried Egg: Top your oatmeal with a perfectly cooked egg for a protein boost.

Cheese: Try grated cheddar or Parmesan for a savory twist.

Fresh Herbs: Add flavor with chopped fresh herbs like chives, cilantro, or parsley.

Sautéed Vegetables: Experiment with sautéed spinach, mushrooms, or cherry tomatoes for a savory oatmeal bowl.

Balanced Toppings:

Greek Yogurt: Creamy Greek yogurt adds protein and creaminess.

Cinnamon: Sprinkle cinnamon for warmth and subtle sweetness.

Dried Fruits: Enhance your oatmeal with dried fruits like raisins, apricots, or cranberries.

Seeds: Chia seeds, flaxseeds, or pumpkin seeds provide added texture and nutrients.

5. Quick and Convenient:

Oatmeal can be prepared in minutes, making it an ideal choice for busy mornings. You can cook it on the stovetop, in the microwave, or even overnight in the fridge for a grab-and-go breakfast.

Oatmeal delight is a versatile, nutritious, and satisfying breakfast option that can suit a variety of tastes and dietary preferences. Whether you're aiming for a sweet, savory, or balanced flavor profile, oatmeal provides a hearty and wholesome base for your favorite toppings and additions. Enjoy the endless possibilities of oatmeal to kickstart your day with a delightful and nourishing meal.

Banana and Honey Oatmeal

Banana and honey oatmeal is a delightful breakfast option that combines the natural sweetness of ripe bananas with the rich, comforting texture of oatmeal. This dish is not only delicious but also packed with essential nutrients, making it a satisfying and wholesome way to start your day. Here's why banana and honey oatmeal are a breakfast delight:

Ingredients:

Oats: Rolled oats or steel-cut oats are the primary base for this dish. They provide fiber, complex carbohydrates, and a creamy texture when cooked.

Bananas: Ripe bananas are the star of the show, adding natural sweetness, creaminess, and essential vitamins like potassium and vitamin C.

Honey: Honey serves as a natural sweetener, adding depth of flavor and a touch of sweetness. It also offers potential health benefits, including antioxidants and antibacterial properties.

Nutritional Benefits:

Fiber: Oats are rich in dietary fiber, which aids digestion, helps maintain stable blood sugar levels, and keeps you feeling full, making it a great choice for weight management.

Potassium: Bananas are a fantastic source of potassium, an essential mineral that supports heart health, muscle function, and electrolyte balance.

Antioxidants: Honey contains antioxidants that can help protect cells from oxidative damage and support overall health.

Satisfaction: The combination of fiber from oats and natural sugars from bananas and honey provides long-lasting energy and keeps hunger at bay.

How to Make Banana and Honey Oatmeal:

Here's a simple recipe to create your own bowl of banana and honey oatmeal:

Ingredients:

1/2 cup rolled oats or steel-cut oats

1 ripe banana, mashed

1 1/2 cups water or milk (dairy or non-dairy)

1-2 tablespoons honey (adjust to taste)

Optional toppings: Sliced bananas, a drizzle of honey, chopped nuts (e.g., almonds, walnuts), a sprinkle of cinnamon, or a dollop of Greek yogurt.

Instructions:

In a saucepan, combine the oats and water or milk. Over medium-high heat, bring to a boil and then turn down the heat.

Simmer the oats, stirring occasionally, for about 5-7 minutes (or according to the package instructions) until they reach your desired level of creaminess.

Stir in the mashed banana and cook for an additional 2-3 minutes, allowing the banana to blend with the oats.

Remove the saucepan from heat and stir in honey to sweeten the oatmeal to your taste. Adjust the amount as needed.

Serve your banana and honey oatmeal in a bowl and add any optional toppings you desire.

Customization:

Feel free to customize your banana and honey oatmeal to suit your preferences. You can adjust the sweetness with more or less honey, add a sprinkle of cinnamon for extra flavor, or experiment with various toppings like chopped nuts, dried fruits, or a dollop of Greek yogurt.

Banana and honey oatmeal are a warm and comforting breakfast that combines the natural sweetness of bananas with the rich creaminess of oatmeal. It's a nutritious and satisfying way to start your day, providing you with essential nutrients, energy, and a comforting taste that's sure to delight your taste buds. Enjoy this wholesome breakfast treat whenever you're in the mood for a sweet and nourishing morning meal.

Almond Butter and Berry Porridge

Almond butter and berry porridge are a delightful and nutritious breakfast option that combines the richness of almond butter with the vibrant flavors of fresh or frozen berries. This comforting dish not only provides a burst of taste but also offers essential nutrients, making it a nourishing and satisfying way to kickstart your day. Here's why almond butter and berry porridge is a breakfast bliss:

Ingredients:

Oats: Rolled oats or steel-cut oats serve as the hearty base for this dish. They provide fiber, complex carbohydrates, and a creamy texture when cooked.

Almond Butter: Almond butter adds creaminess and a nutty flavor while providing healthy fats, protein, and vitamin E.

Berries: Fresh or frozen berries (such as strawberries, blueberries, raspberries, or blackberries) bring natural sweetness, vibrant colors, and a dose of antioxidants to the porridge.

Honey (optional): Honey can serve as a natural sweetener, enhancing the overall flavor profile and offering potential health benefits, including antioxidants and antibacterial properties.

Nutritional Benefits:

Fiber: Oats are a fantastic source of dietary fiber, which supports healthy digestion, helps maintain stable blood sugar levels, and keeps you feeling full, aiding in weight management.

Healthy Fats: Almond butter provides monounsaturated fats, which are heart-healthy and may help reduce the risk of heart disease.

Protein: Almond butter also contributes to the protein content of the dish, helping to keep you satisfied and supporting muscle maintenance and repair.

Antioxidants: Berries are rich in antioxidants, which can help protect cells from oxidative damage and promote overall health.

Vitamins and Minerals: Berries are a source of essential vitamins like vitamin C and vitamin K, as well as minerals like potassium and manganese.

How to Make Almond Butter and Berry Porridge:

Here's a simple recipe to create your own bowl of almond butter and berry porridge:

Ingredients:

1/2 cup rolled oats or steel-cut oats

1 1/2 cups water or milk (dairy or non-dairy)

2 tablespoons almond butter

1/2 cup fresh or frozen mixed berries

Optional sweetener: 1-2 tablespoons honey or maple syrup, to taste

Optional toppings: Sliced almonds, a drizzle of almond butter, additional berries, or a sprinkle of cinnamon.

Instructions:

In a saucepan, combine the oats and water or milk. Turn the heat down to low after bringing to a boil over medium-high heat.

Simmer the oats, stirring occasionally, for about 5-7 minutes (or according to the package instructions) until they reach your desired level of creaminess.

Stir in the almond butter until it's well incorporated with the oatmeal.

Add the mixed berries and continue to cook for an additional 2-3 minutes, allowing the berries to heat through.

If desired, sweeten your porridge with honey or maple syrup to taste.

Serve your almond butter and berry porridge in a bowl and add any optional toppings you prefer.

Customization:

Feel free to customize your almond butter and berry porridge according to your preferences. Adjust the sweetness, texture, or toppings to suit your taste. You can also experiment with different types of berries or nut butters for variety.

Almond butter and berry porridge is a nutritious and flavorful breakfast that combines the creamy richness of almond butter with the vibrant freshness of berries. It's a wholesome and satisfying way to start your day, providing you with essential nutrients, energy, and a burst of delicious flavors that will leave you craving more. Enjoy this delightful breakfast creation whenever you want a nourishing and comforting morning meal.

Smoothie Sensations

Smoothies have become a beloved breakfast and snack option for those seeking both convenience and nutrition. These blended concoctions, often referred to as "Smoothie Sensations," are packed with an array of wholesome ingredients that not only tantalize your taste buds but also provide your body with essential nutrients. Let's explore why smoothies have gained popularity and how you can create your own smoothie sensations:

Why Smoothies Are Sensational:

Nutrient Density: Smoothies offer a convenient way to pack a variety of nutrient-dense ingredients into one delicious drink. You can load them up with fruits, vegetables, nuts, seeds, and more, providing a wide range of vitamins, minerals, and antioxidants.

Quick and Easy: Preparing a smoothie takes only minutes, making it an ideal option for busy mornings or a healthy on-the-go snack.

Customization: The beauty of smoothies lies in their versatility. You can customize your smoothie to suit your taste preferences, dietary needs, and specific health goals.

Hydration: Many smoothie ingredients, such as fruits and vegetables, have a high-water content, helping you stay hydrated.

Digestibility: Blending breaks down food into a more digestible form, making it easier for your body to absorb nutrients.

Building Blocks for a Sensational Smoothie:
To create your own smoothie sensations, start with these basic building blocks:

Base Liquid: Choose a liquid as the foundation for your smoothie. Options include water, milk (dairy or non-dairy like almond, soy, or oat milk), yogurt, or even green tea for an antioxidant boost.

Fruits and Vegetables: Incorporate a mix of fruits and vegetables for flavor and nutrition. Common choices include bananas, berries, spinach, kale, avocado, and cucumber. Frozen fruits can add a creamy texture and keep your smoothie cold.

Protein: Add protein to make your smoothie more satisfying and support muscle repair and growth. Options include Greek yogurt, protein powder, tofu, or nut butter.

Healthy Fats: Include sources of healthy fats like avocados, nuts (e.g., almonds, walnuts), seeds (e.g., chia, flax, or hemp seeds), or a spoonful of coconut oil. These fats contribute to satiety and provide essential fatty acids.

Sweeteners (Optional): If you prefer a sweeter smoothie, add natural sweeteners like honey, maple syrup, or dates. Be mindful of added sugars and use these sweeteners sparingly.

Extras: Boost your smoothie with extra nutrients by adding ingredients like greens (e.g., spinach, kale), spices (e.g., cinnamon, turmeric), or superfood powders (e.g., spirulina, maca).

Smoothie Sensation Recipes:

Here are a few delightful smoothie sensation recipes to get you started:

1. Berry Blast Smoothie:

1 cup mixed berries (strawberries, blueberries, raspberries)

1/2 banana

1/2 cup Greek yogurt

1 tablespoon honey

1 cup almond milk

2. Green Goddess Smoothie:

1 cup spinach

1/2 avocado

1/2 banana

1 tablespoon chia seeds

1 cup coconut water

3. Peanut Butter Power Smoothie:

2 tablespoons peanut butter

1 banana

1/4 cup oats

1 cup milk (dairy or non-dairy)

A drizzle of honey

4. Tropical Paradise Smoothie:

1/2 cup pineapple chunks

1/2 cup mango chunks

1/2 cup Greek yogurt

1 tablespoon coconut oil

1 cup coconut milk

You can experiment with flavors, textures, and ingredients while providing your body with necessary nutrients by making your own smoothie creations. Smoothies offer a delicious way to delight your palate and nourish your body for the day ahead, whether you're searching for a quick breakfast, a post-workout snack, or a nutritious indulgence. Use your imagination, combine your preferred ingredients, and savor the lovely world of smoothie delights!

Papaya and Ginger Smoothie

A papaya and ginger smoothie are a tropical delight that combines the sweet, vibrant flavors of papaya with the zesty kick of fresh ginger. This refreshing and nutrient-packed concoction not only invigorates your taste buds but also provides numerous health benefits. Here's why a papaya and ginger smoothie are fantastic addition to your culinary repertoire:

Nutritional Powerhouse:

Papaya: This tropical fruit is a nutritional treasure trove, rich in vitamins (particularly vitamin C and vitamin A), dietary fiber, and a variety of antioxidants. Papaya is also known for its enzyme called papain, which aids digestion.

Ginger: Ginger is well known for its digestive and anti-inflammatory qualities. It contains gingerol, a bioactive compound with potential health benefits, such as reducing nausea and easing muscle pain.

Protein: Depending on your preference, you can add protein sources like Greek yogurt, almond milk, or a protein powder of your choice to make your smoothie more satisfying.

Fiber: Papaya and ginger both contribute dietary fiber, which supports digestive health and helps keep you feeling full.

Health Benefits:

Digestive Aid: Ginger is well-known for its ability to alleviate digestive discomfort, reduce nausea, and ease indigestion. Combined with papaya's natural enzymes, this smoothie is gentle on the stomach.

Anti-Inflammatory: Ginger contains potent anti-inflammatory compounds that may help reduce inflammation and support overall health.

Immune Boost: The high vitamin C content in papaya can boost your immune system, potentially helping to ward off illnesses.

Hydration: Papaya has a high-water content, contributing to hydration, and ginger can help alleviate dehydration-related symptoms like nausea.

How to Make a Papaya and Ginger Smoothie:

Here's a simple recipe to create your own papaya and ginger smoothie:

Ingredients:

1 cup ripe papaya, diced

1 small piece of fresh ginger (about 1 inch), peeled and minced

1/2 cup Greek yogurt or non-dairy yogurt

1/2 cup of almond milk, or any other type of milk

1-2 tablespoons of honey (optional, for extra sweetness) or maple syrup

A handful of ice cubes (optional)

Instructions:

Place all the ingredients in a blender.

Blend until smooth and creamy. To get the right consistency, you can add extra milk if the smoothie is too thick.

After tasting the smoothie, taste it again and add more honey or maple syrup if needed to make it sweeter.

Pour your papaya and ginger smoothie into a glass and enjoy immediately.

Customization:

Feel free to customize your papaya and ginger smoothie to suit your preferences:

Add a banana for extra creaminess and natural sweetness.

Include a handful of spinach or kale for added nutrients without altering the flavor significantly.

Add a dollop of nut butter or a scoop of your preferred protein powder to increase the protein content.

A papaya and ginger smoothie is a refreshing and nutritious way to start your day or enjoy as a midday snack. Its combination of tropical sweetness and zesty ginger creates a harmonious flavor profile, while the health benefits of these ingredients make it a sensible choice for overall well-being. Whether you're sipping it for its digestive properties or simply for its delightful taste, this smoothie is a true tropical sensation.

Spinach and Banana Green Smoothie

A spinach and banana green smoothie is a vibrant and nutritious concoction that combines the earthy goodness of spinach with the natural sweetness of ripe bananas. This emerald elixir not only tantalizes your taste buds but also provides your body with essential nutrients, making it a refreshing and healthful way to start your day. Here's why a spinach and banana green smoothie is a fantastic addition to your daily routine:

Nutritional Powerhouse:

Spinach: Spinach is a nutritional powerhouse, loaded with vitamins (especially vitamin K, vitamin A, and folate), minerals (such as iron and potassium), and dietary fiber. It's also rich in antioxidants, which help protect your cells from damage.

Bananas: Bananas give the smoothie a naturally sweet and creamy texture. They are a great source of dietary fibre, potassium, and vitamin B6.

Protein: Depending on your preference, you can enhance the protein content of your smoothie by adding Greek yogurt, almond milk, or a scoop of protein powder.

Fiber: Spinach and bananas both contribute to the dietary fiber content, which supports digestion and helps keep you feeling full.

Health Benefits:
Nutrient Density: Spinach is low in calories but high in nutrients, making it an excellent choice for a nutrient-dense breakfast or snack.

Digestive Health: The fiber in spinach aids digestion, while the natural sugars in bananas help regulate bowel movements.

Potassium: Both spinach and bananas are rich in potassium, which supports heart health and helps regulate blood pressure.

Antioxidants: Spinach is a source of powerful antioxidants like lutein and zeaxanthin, which are beneficial for eye health.

Energy Boost: The natural sugars and carbohydrates in bananas provide a quick and sustainable source of energy.

How to Make a Spinach and Banana Green Smoothie:

Here's a simple recipe to create your own spinach and banana green smoothie:

Ingredients:

1 cup fresh spinach leaves (or frozen, if preferred)

1 ripe banana

1/2 cup Greek yogurt or non-dairy yogurt

1/2 cup of your preferred milk, or almond milk

1-2 teaspoons of maple syrup or honey (optional, for added

A handful of ice cubes (optional)

Instructions:

Place all the ingredients in a blender.

Blend until smooth and creamy. To get the right consistency, you can add extra milk if the smoothie is too thick.

After tasting the smoothie, taste it again and add more honey or maple syrup if needed to make it sweeter.

Pour your spinach and banana green smoothie into a glass and enjoy immediately.

Customization:

Feel free to customize your spinach and banana green smoothie to suit your preferences:

Add a scoop of protein powder to boost the protein content for a post-workout snack.

Include a tablespoon of flaxseeds or chia seeds for added fiber and healthy fats.

Experiment with different greens like kale, Swiss chard, or arugula for variety.

A spinach and banana green smoothie is a refreshing and nutrient-packed way to fuel your body with essential vitamins and minerals. Its combination of leafy greens and naturally sweet bananas creates a harmonious flavor profile that's both delicious and healthful. Whether you're sipping it for its nutrient density, energy boost, or simply for its delightful taste, this smoothie is a green elixir of health that can help you stay nourished and energized throughout the day.

Breakfast Quiches and Omelets

Breakfast quiches and omelets are savory breakfast dishes that have become popular choices for those seeking a hearty and protein-packed start to their day. Both options offer endless possibilities for creativity in the kitchen, allowing you to personalize your morning meal to your taste preferences and dietary needs. Here's a closer look at breakfast quiches and omelets, why they're so beloved, and how you can create your own delightful variations.

Breakfast Quiches:

A breakfast quiche is a savory pie made with a pastry crust filled with a mixture of eggs, cream or milk, cheese, and a variety of ingredients such as vegetables, meats, and herbs. Here's what makes quiches stand out:

Versatility: Breakfast quiches can be customized with a wide range of ingredients, making them suitable for different dietary preferences. Common additions include spinach, mushrooms, bell peppers, bacon, ham, and various types of cheese.

Protein-Rich: Eggs are the star of the show in quiches, providing a protein-packed base that helps keep you satisfied throughout the morning.

Flavor Profile: The combination of ingredients in a quiche creates a harmonious blend of flavors, and the golden-brown crust adds a delightful textural contrast.

Make-Ahead: Quiches can be prepared in advance, making them a convenient option for busy mornings. You can store them in the refrigerator and reheat slices as needed.

Omelets:
Omelets are a classic breakfast choice that consists of beaten eggs cooked in a skillet and filled with a variety of ingredients. Here's why omelets are a beloved morning staple:

Quick and Customizable: Omelets can be made in a matter of minutes, making them perfect for busy mornings. You can personalize them with your favorite ingredients, such as cheese, vegetables, herbs, and meats.

Protein-Packed: Eggs provide a substantial amount of protein, making omelets a satisfying and nourishing breakfast option.

Low in Carbs: Omelets are naturally low in carbohydrates, making them suitable for those following low-carb or keto diets.

Healthy Fats: You can add healthy fats like avocado or olive oil to boost flavor and nutritional value.

Texture and Flavor: The combination of creamy eggs and various fillings creates a delightful contrast in both texture and flavor.

Creating Your Own Breakfast Quiches and Omelets:
Here are some tips for crafting your own breakfast quiches and omelets:

For Quiches:
Choose Your Crust: You can use a traditional pastry crust, a potato crust, or a crustless option for a lower-carb alternative.

Select Your Fillings: Combine ingredients like sautéed vegetables, cooked meats, and grated cheese. Be sure to pre-cook any ingredients that release excess moisture to prevent a soggy crust.

Whisk Eggs: In a separate bowl, whisk eggs with cream or milk, salt, pepper, and any desired herbs or spices.

Assemble: Layer the fillings in the prepared crust and pour the egg mixture over them.

Bake: Bake your quiche until it's set and golden brown.

For Omelets:

Beat Eggs: Whisk eggs in a bowl until well combined. Add salt and pepper to taste.

Preheat Pan: Heat a non-stick skillet over medium-high heat and add a small amount of butter or oil.

Add Fillings: Pour the beaten eggs into the skillet and let them set slightly. Place the fillings of your choice on half of the omelets.

Fold and Serve: Once the eggs are mostly set, fold the other half of the omelets over the fillings. After sliding it onto a dish, serve.

Whether you choose a breakfast quiche or omelets, both options offer a delightful combination of flavors and the flexibility to suit your dietary preferences. With endless possibilities for customization, you can create morning dishes that satisfy your cravings and provide the fuel you need to start your day on the right foot.

Veggie and Turkey Quiche

Veggie and turkey quiche are a savory breakfast dish that brings together the goodness of vegetables, lean turkey, and a creamy egg filling baked in a flaky crust. This delightful quiche not only offers a burst of flavors but also provides a range of essential nutrients, making it a wholesome and satisfying way to begin your day. Here's why veggie and turkey quiche are fantastic addition to your breakfast repertoire:

Nutritional Powerhouse:
Lean Protein: Turkey is a lean source of protein, which supports muscle health and helps keep you feeling full.

Vitamins and Minerals: The vegetables in this quiche contribute essential vitamins (such as vitamin A, vitamin C, and vitamin K) and minerals (including potassium, folate, and magnesium).

Fiber: Vegetables like spinach and bell peppers add dietary fiber to the quiche, aiding in digestion and promoting satiety.

Healthy Fats: Eggs and dairy ingredients in the quiche provide healthy fats that are essential for overall health.

Flavorful Ingredients:
Turkey: Lean ground turkey or turkey sausage adds a savory and mildly seasoned flavor to the quiche, creating a satisfying balance with the vegetables.

Vegetables: Common choices include spinach, bell peppers, onions, and mushrooms. These ingredients contribute a variety of textures and tastes to the quiche.

Cheese: A generous amount of cheese, such as cheddar, Swiss, or feta, adds creaminess and enhances the overall flavor profile.

Eggs: The creamy egg filling binds all the ingredients together and provides a rich and indulgent texture.

How to Make Veggie and Turkey Quiche:

Here's a simple recipe to create your own veggie and turkey quiche:

Ingredients:

1 pie crust (store-bought or homemade)

1/2-pound lean ground turkey or turkey sausage

1 cup fresh spinach leaves, chopped

1/2 cup finely chopped bell peppers (red or green)

1/2 cup onion, finely chopped

1/2 cup mushrooms, sliced

1 1/2 cups shredded cheese (cheddar, Swiss, or your choice)

4 large eggs

1 cup milk (dairy or non-dairy)

Salt and pepper to taste

Olive oil for sautéing

Instructions:

Preheat your oven to 375°F (190°C).

In a skillet, heat a small amount of olive oil over medium-high heat. Add the ground turkey or turkey sausage and cook until browned. Remove any excess fat.

In the same skillet, add a bit more oil if needed, then sauté the onions, bell peppers, and mushrooms until they are tender.

Place the pie crust in a greased pie dish.

Layer the cooked turkey and sautéed vegetables in the pie crust, then sprinkle the shredded cheese on top.

Beat the eggs, milk, pepper, and salt in another bowl.

Pour this mixture over the turkey, vegetables, and cheese in the pie crust.

Bake for 35 to 40 minutes, or until the quiche is set and the top is browned. Preheat the oven.

Prior to slicing and serving, let the quiche cool slightly.

Customization:

Feel free to customize your veggie and turkey quiche to suit your preferences. You can:

Add herbs like thyme, rosemary, or basil for extra flavor.

Use a mix of cheeses or a different kind of cheese.

Swap out the vegetables for your favorites or based on what's in season.

Veggie and turkey quiche is a flavorful and nutrient-packed breakfast option that combines the savory goodness of lean turkey, an array of vegetables, and a creamy egg filling. It's a wholesome and satisfying way to start your day, providing you with essential nutrients, protein, and a delightful combination of flavors and textures. Enjoy this savory breakfast delight as a family favorite or make it in advance for a convenient grab-and-go morning meal.

Spinach and Feta Omelets

A spinach and feta omelets are a Mediterranean-inspired breakfast that combines the earthy flavor of spinach with the creamy, tangy goodness of feta cheese. This savory omelet not only tantalizes your taste buds but also provides a range of essential nutrients, making it a wholesome and satisfying way to kickstart your day. Here's why a spinach and feta omelet is a fantastic addition to your breakfast rotation:

Nutritional Powerhouse:

Spinach: Spinach is a nutritional gem, packed with vitamins (especially vitamin K, vitamin A, and folate), minerals (including iron and potassium), and dietary fiber. It's also rich in antioxidants like lutein and zeaxanthin, which are beneficial for eye health.

Feta Cheese: Feta cheese adds creaminess and a tangy kick to the omelet while providing protein, calcium, and healthy fats.

Protein: Eggs are the star of the show in omelets, providing a protein-packed base that helps keep you satisfied throughout the morning.

Healthy Fats: The combination of eggs and feta cheese contributes healthy fats, which are essential for overall health and satiety.

Flavorful Ingredients:

Spinach: Fresh spinach leaves bring an earthy and slightly bitter flavor that pairs beautifully with the creaminess of the eggs and feta.

Feta Cheese: Feta's tangy and salty profile contrasts with the mildness of the spinach, adding depth of flavor to the omelet.

Eggs: Eggs create a rich and creamy texture while providing protein and essential nutrients.

Herbs and Seasonings: Optional additions like fresh herbs (e.g., parsley or dill), black pepper, and a pinch of nutmeg can elevate the flavor profile.

How to Make a Spinach and Feta Omelets:

Here's a simple recipe to create your own spinach and feta omelet:

Ingredients:

2 large eggs

1/2 cup fresh spinach leaves, roughly chopped

2 tablespoons crumbled feta cheese

Salt and pepper to taste

A dash of nutmeg (optional)

Cooking oil or butter for the pan

Instructions:

Crack the eggs into a bowl, add a pinch of salt and pepper, and whisk until well beaten. You can also add a dash of nutmeg at this stage if desired.

Heat a non-stick skillet over medium-high heat and add a small amount of cooking oil or butter to coat the bottom.

Once the skillet is hot, add the chopped spinach leaves and sauté for about 1-2 minutes until they start to wilt.

Pour the beaten eggs over the wilted spinach and let them cook undisturbed for a minute or so until the edges start to set.

Sprinkle the crumbled feta cheese evenly over one-half of the omelet.

Gently lift the other half of the omelet with a spatula and fold it over the cheese side to create a half-moon shape.

Cook for an additional minute or until the eggs are fully set and the cheese is slightly melted.

Carefully slide the spinach and feta omelet onto a plate, season with additional salt and pepper if desired, and garnish with fresh herbs if available.

Customization:

Feel free to customize your spinach and feta omelet to suit your preferences:

Add diced tomatoes or sun-dried tomatoes for a burst of freshness and color.

Include a pinch of red pepper flakes for a touch of heat.

Experiment with different herbs and spices to create unique flavor profiles.

A spinach and feta omelets are a flavorful and nutrient-packed breakfast option that celebrates the Mediterranean diet's delicious and wholesome ingredients. Whether you're savoring it as a leisurely weekend breakfast or whipping it up for a quick and nutritious weekday meal, this omelet is a delightful way to start your day with a burst of flavor and nutrition.

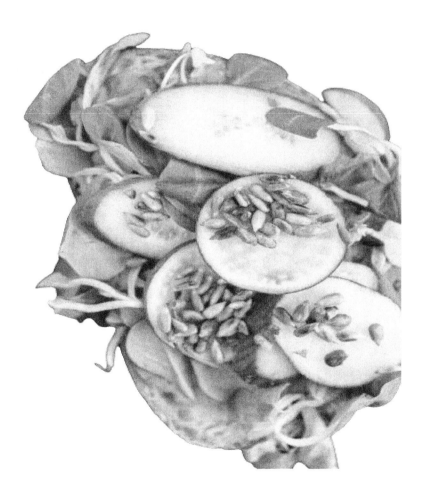

Chapter 3

Nourishing Lunches and Light Dinners

Nourishing lunches and light dinners are essential components of a balanced daily diet. These meals play a crucial role in providing you with the energy and nutrients you need to maintain optimal health and well-being. Let's explore the benefits of each and how you can make the most of them in your daily eating routine.

Nourishing Lunches:

A nourishing lunch is the cornerstone of your midday meal, serving as a source of sustenance and fuel to power you through the rest of your day. Here are some key reasons why nourishing lunches are important:

Energy Boost: Lunch replenishes your energy levels after a morning of activity. It helps you stay alert and focused in the afternoon.

Nutrient Intake: Lunch offers an opportunity to consume a variety of nutrients, including vitamins, minerals, protein, and healthy fats. A well-balanced lunch can support overall health and well-being.

Satiety: A satisfying lunch helps prevent excessive snacking between meals, which can be beneficial for weight management.

Digestive Break: Eating a substantial lunch allows your digestive system to process food during its most active hours, which can improve digestion and reduce discomfort.

Tips for Nourishing Lunches:

Include a balance of macronutrients: Incorporate protein (e.g., lean meats, poultry, fish, tofu, beans), carbohydrates (e.g., whole grains, fruits, vegetables), and healthy fats (e.g., avocados, nuts, olive oil) to create a satisfying and nutritious meal.

Opt for fiber-rich foods: Foods like vegetables, whole grains, and legumes provide dietary fiber, which supports digestive health and helps keep you full.

Portion control: Pay attention to portion proportions to prevent overindulging. Listen to your body's hunger cues.

Meal prep: Preparing your lunch in advance can help you make healthier choices and save time during busy workdays.

Light Dinners:

A light dinner serves as the closing act of your day, providing nourishment without overwhelming your digestive system before bedtime. Here's why light dinners are essential:

Digestive Comfort: A light dinner allows your digestive system to wind down, promoting better sleep and reducing the risk of discomfort like heartburn or indigestion.

Weight Management: Eating a smaller, lighter dinner can contribute to better weight management since it gives your body less time to store calories as fat before bedtime.

Quality Sleep: A lighter dinner can support more restful sleep, as heavy or rich foods late at night can disrupt sleep patterns.

Balanced Intake: By having a substantial lunch and a lighter dinner, you ensure that your body receives the necessary nutrients throughout the day without excessive calorie intake in the evening.

Tips for Light Dinners:

Opt for lean proteins: Include sources like grilled chicken, fish, or plant-based proteins like tofu or legumes.

Emphasize vegetables: Load up on veggies for fiber, vitamins, and minerals. A salad or roasted vegetables can be a great foundation for a light dinner.

Minimize heavy sauces and fried foods: Avoid rich, heavy, or fried dishes that may be harder to digest in the evening.

Control portion sizes: Keep dinner portions moderate to prevent overeating and promote better digestion.

Time your dinner wisely: Aim to finish dinner at least two to three hours before bedtime to allow for proper digestion.

By embracing nourishing lunches and light dinners, you can strike a balance in your daily nutrition, supporting your energy levels, overall health, and well-being. These meals play complementary roles in your daily diet, providing the sustenance you need during active hours and the digestive comfort required for restful sleep. Remember to focus on balanced and wholesome food choices while listening to your body's hunger cues to make the most of these important meals in your daily routine.

Hearty Soups

Hearty soups are the epitome of comfort food, offering warmth, nourishment, and a symphony of flavors in every spoonful. These soul-soothing concoctions come in various forms and are enjoyed around the world, providing both sustenance and a sense of comfort. Let's explore why hearty soups hold a special place in culinary traditions and how they can be a versatile and nourishing addition to your meals.

What Makes Soups Hearty:

Hearty soups are characterized by several key elements:

Substantial Ingredients: They typically contain substantial ingredients like vegetables, legumes, grains, meats, or seafood, which add texture and substance to the soup.

Rich Broths: Hearty soups often feature flavorful broths or stocks that provide a robust and satisfying base. These broths can be made from scratch or enhanced with seasonings and aromatic ingredients.

Variety of Flavors: They incorporate a rich combination of flavors from various ingredients, herbs, and spices, creating a harmonious taste profile.

Filling and Satisfying: Hearty soups are meant to be filling and satisfying, making them suitable as a meal on their own or a substantial course in a larger meal.

Why We Love Hearty Soups:

Comfort and Warmth: Hearty soups provide a comforting feeling, especially on chilly days or when you're in need of a pick-me-up.

Versatility: They are incredibly versatile, allowing you to use ingredients you have on hand to create delicious, one-pot meals.

Nutrient Density: Soups often contain a medley of vegetables and proteins, making them a nutrient-dense option for getting essential vitamins and minerals.

Ease of Preparation: Most hearty soups are simple to prepare, requiring minimal hands-on time, making them accessible for home cooks of all levels.

Popular Types of Hearty Soups:

Minestrone: An Italian classic, minestrone features a tomato-based broth with a variety of vegetables, beans, and pasta.

Chili: This Tex-Mex favorite combine's ground meat (usually beef) with beans, tomatoes, and spices, resulting in a hearty and spicy soup.

Chicken Noodle: A comforting classic, chicken noodle soup is made with chicken, vegetables, and noodles in a savory broth.

Lentil Soup: Lentil soups are hearty and rich in plant-based protein, often flavored with aromatic spices like cumin and coriander.

Split Pea Soup: Made from split peas, this soup has a thick and creamy texture and is typically flavored with ham or bacon.

Beef Stew: A slow-cooked favorite, beef stew features tender chunks of beef, root vegetables, and a savory broth.

Tips for Making Hearty Soups:

Use a flavorful base: Start with a flavorful broth or stock to build the foundation of your soup.

Layer your ingredients: Add ingredients in stages, allowing each component to contribute to the overall flavor.

Experiment with herbs and spices: Fresh herbs and aromatic spices can elevate the taste of your soup.

Don't rush: Many hearty soups benefit from slow simmering, which allows flavors to meld and intensify.

Hearty soups are more than just a meal; they are a comforting and nourishing experience. Whether you're seeking warmth on a cold day, a satisfying and nutritious meal, or simply the joy of savoring different flavors, hearty soups offer a culinary journey that satisfies the senses and warms the heart. So, grab a ladle, embrace the comfort of a hearty bowl of soup, and savor the delightful world of flavors that these comforting dishes bring to your table.

Chicken and Rice Soup

Chicken and rice soup are a beloved and timeless classic that combines tender pieces of chicken, aromatic vegetables, flavorful broth, and rice into a hearty and comforting bowl of goodness. This soul-soothing soup is cherished for its nourishing qualities and the way it warms both body and soul, making it a favorite in kitchens around the world. Let's explore what makes chicken and rice soup so special and how to make a delicious batch for yourself.

Key Ingredients:

Chicken: Chicken is the star of the show in this soup. You can use bone-in chicken pieces, boneless chicken breasts or thighs, or even leftover roasted chicken. It provides lean protein and a mild, savory flavor.

Rice: White or brown rice adds heartiness to the soup and makes it a filling meal. Rice grains absorb the flavorful broth as they cook, infusing the soup with a satisfying texture.

Vegetables: A medley of vegetables like carrots, celery, and onions lend a rich flavor base and provide essential vitamins and minerals.

Broth: Chicken broth or stock forms the flavorful foundation of the soup. Homemade broth is ideal, but store-bought options work well too.

Herbs and Spices: Common additions include bay leaves, thyme, parsley, and black pepper, which enhance the soup's aroma and taste.

Why We Love Chicken and Rice Soup:

Comforting Warmth: A bowl of chicken and rice soup is like a warm hug, perfect for comforting you on chilly days or when you're feeling under the weather.

Versatile and Filling: This soup is highly versatile. You can customize it with your favorite vegetables, herbs, or spices to suit your taste. It's also filling enough to be a standalone meal.

Nutrient-Rich: It's packed with nutrients from the chicken, vegetables, and broth, making it a wholesome choice for a balanced diet.

Ease of Preparation: Chicken and rice soup is straightforward to make, and it's an excellent way to use up leftover chicken.

How to Make Chicken and Rice Soup:

Here's a basic recipe for homemade chicken and rice soup:

Ingredients:

2 boneless, skinless chicken breasts, or 1 pound of bone-in chicken pieces

1 cup rice (white or brown)

2 carrots, peeled and diced

2 celery stalks, diced

1 onion, finely chopped

6 cups chicken broth

2 bay leaves

1 teaspoon dried thyme

Salt and black pepper to taste

Fresh parsley for garnish

Olive oil for sautéing

Instructions:

Heat a sprinkle of olive oil in a big pot over medium heat.

Add the chopped onion, carrots, and celery. Sauté for 5-7 minutes until the vegetables start to soften.

Add the chicken breasts or pieces to the pot and cook for about 5 minutes, or until they are no longer pink on the outside.

Add the dried thyme and bay leaves after adding the chicken broth. Bring the soup to a boil, then reduce the heat to low, cover, and simmer for about 20-25 minutes until the chicken is cooked through.

Remove the chicken from the pot and shred it into bite-sized pieces using two forks. Back in the pot, add the shredded chicken. Stir in the rice and continue to simmer for another 15-20 minutes until the rice is tender.

Add salt and black pepper to taste when preparing the soup. Remove the bay leaves.

Ladle the hot chicken and rice soup into bowls, garnish with fresh parsley, and serve.

Customization:

Feel free to get creative with your chicken and rice soup:

Add extra vegetables like peas, corn, or spinach for additional color and nutrition.

Try a variety of herbs and spices to see what suits your palate best. Make it creamy by stirring in a bit of heavy cream or coconut milk.

If you have leftover cooked chicken, skip the initial cooking step and add the shredded chicken when you add the rice.

Chicken and rice soup is a classic comfort food that's nourishing, flavorful, and endlessly adaptable to your preferences. Whether you're craving a bowl of warmth on a cold day or a soothing meal to comfort your soul, this timeless Soup is a certain way to sate your appetite and make your table feel cozy.

Creamy Butternut Squash Soup

Creamy butternut squash soup is a luxurious and velvety concoction that embodies the rich, sweet, and nutty flavors of butternut squash. This soup is a beloved fall and winter classic, celebrated for its comforting warmth, delightful aroma, and satisfying creaminess. Whether you enjoy it as a cozy appetizer or a hearty meal, here's why creamy butternut squash soup is a culinary masterpiece and how to make your own bowl of this delightful comfort food.

Key Ingredients:

Butternut Squash: The star ingredient, butternut squash, is known for its vibrant orange flesh and slightly sweet, nutty flavor. It's high in fibre, antioxidants, and vitamins A and C.

Onion and Garlic: These aromatics provide depth of flavor to the soup.

Broth: Chicken or vegetable broth forms the base of the soup, infusing it with savory notes. You can use homemade or store-bought broth.

Cream or Coconut Milk: To achieve the creamy texture, you can opt for heavy cream, half-and-half, or coconut milk (for a dairy-free version).

Spices: Common spices include nutmeg, cinnamon, and a pinch of cayenne for a subtle kick.

Why We Love Creamy Butternut Squash Soup:

Warmth and Comfort: Creamy butternut squash soup offers warmth and comfort, making it a perfect choice on cold days or when you need a cozy, soul-soothing meal.

Flavor Complexity: It boasts a harmonious blend of sweet, savory, and slightly earthy flavors, making it a sophisticated yet approachable dish.

Versatility: You can customize the soup to suit your taste by adjusting the level of sweetness, creaminess, or spice to your liking.

Nutrient-Rich: Butternut squash is a nutrient powerhouse, packed with vitamins, minerals, and fiber. This soup allows you to enjoy these health benefits in a delicious way.

How to Make Creamy Butternut Squash Soup:

Here's a basic recipe to create your own creamy butternut squash soup:

Ingredients:

1 medium butternut squash (about 4 cups), peeled, seeds, and cubed

1 onion, chopped

2 cloves garlic, minced

4 cups chicken or vegetable broth

1 cup heavy cream or coconut milk

1/2 teaspoon ground nutmeg

1/4 teaspoon ground cinnamon

Pinch of cayenne pepper (optional)

Salt and black pepper to taste

Olive oil for sautéing

Fresh parsley or chives for garnish (optional)

Instructions:

Heat a sprinkle of olive oil in a big pot over medium heat. Add the chopped onion and garlic and sauté for about 3-5 minutes until softened.

Add the cubed butternut squash and continue to cook for another 5 minutes, stirring occasionally.

Pour in the chicken or vegetable broth, ensuring that it covers the squash. Bring the mixture to a boil, then reduce the heat to low, cover, and simmer for about 20-25 minutes, or until the squash is fork-tender.

After taking the pot from the stove, let it to cool somewhat. Puree the soup with an immersion blender until it's smooth. If you don't have an immersion blender, you can use a countertop blender in batches.

Transfer the pureed soup back into the pot and set it on a low burner. Stir in the heavy cream or coconut milk, nutmeg, cinnamon, and cayenne pepper (if using). To taste, add salt and black pepper for seasoning.

Allow the soup to heat through without boiling, stirring gently.

Ladle the creamy butternut squash soup into bowls, garnish with fresh parsley or chives if desired, and serve hot.

Customization:

For added depth of flavor, you can roast the cubed butternut squash in the oven before adding it to the soup.

Adjust the level of creaminess by adding more or less heavy cream or coconut milk.

Experiment with different spices and herbs to create unique flavor profiles, such as sage or thyme.

Creamy butternut squash soup is a culinary masterpiece that captures the essence of fall and winter in every spoonful. Its velvety texture, harmonious flavors, and versatility make it a delightful addition to your seasonal menu. Whether you savor it as an appetizer, side dish, or a nourishing meal on its own, this soup is sure to warm your heart and satisfy your taste buds.

Salad Creations

Salad creations are a delightful journey into the world of fresh ingredients, vibrant colors, and tantalizing flavors. These culinary masterpieces allow you to express your creativity in the kitchen while embracing a healthy and nutritious lifestyle. Whether you're a seasoned chef or a novice home cook, crafting your salad creation is an art form that can satisfy your taste buds and nourish your body. Let's dive into the world of salad creations and discover what makes them so special.

The Canvas: Fresh and Wholesome Ingredients

At the heart of every salad creation are fresh and wholesome ingredients. These ingredients serve as the canvas on which you'll paint your culinary masterpiece. Here are some key elements:

Greens: Start with a bed of fresh greens like lettuce, spinach, arugula, or kale. These provide a nutrient-rich base for your salad.

Vegetables: Add a rainbow of vegetables, such as tomatoes, cucumbers, bell peppers, carrots, and radishes. These provide color, crunch, and essential vitamins.

Proteins: Incorporate proteins like grilled chicken, tofu, chickpeas, or beans for a satisfying and filling salad.

Fruits: Fresh or dried fruits like berries, apples, oranges, or figs can add sweetness and a burst of flavor.

Nuts and Seeds: Toasted almonds, walnuts, pumpkin seeds, or sunflower seeds offer texture and a delightful crunch.

Cheese: A sprinkle of cheese, such as feta, goat cheese, or Parmesan, can add creaminess and umami.

Dressing: Choose a dressing that complements your ingredients, whether it's a classic vinaigrette, creamy ranch, or a balsamic glaze.

The Artistry: Creating Your Salad

Creating a salad is not just about tossing ingredients together; it's an art form that involves balance, contrast, and harmony. Here are some tips to help you create a salad masterpiece:

Balance Textures: Combine ingredients with different textures, such as crisp vegetables, tender greens, crunchy nuts, and chewy dried fruits.

Mix Colors: Aim for a vibrant color palette in your salad to make it visually appealing. Different colors often signify different nutrients.

Flavor Harmony: Balance flavors by combining sweet and savory elements, acidic and creamy components, and mild and bold tastes.

Protein Choice: Select proteins that complement your salad's theme. For example, grilled shrimp for a Mediterranean salad or grilled steak for a hearty steakhouse salad.

Dressing Drizzle: Dress your salad just before serving to prevent wilting. Use restraint with dressing; a little goes a long way.

Layering: Consider layering your ingredients for a visually appealing presentation. Start with greens on the bottom and arrange other ingredients on top.

Endless Possibilities: Salad Inspirations

Salad creations offer endless possibilities, inspired by cuisines from around the world and seasonal ingredients. Here are some salad inspirations to get your creative juices flowing:

Greek Salad: Tomatoes, cucumbers, Kalamata olives, red onions, and feta cheese with a lemon-oregano vinaigrette.

Cobb Salad: Lettuce, grilled chicken, bacon, hard-boiled eggs, avocado, tomatoes, and blue cheese dressing.

Caprese Salad: Fresh mozzarella, tomatoes, and basil leaves drizzled with balsamic glaze and olive oil.

Asian-Inspired Salad: Napa cabbage, shredded carrots, edamame, grilled tofu, and sesame ginger dressing.

Fruit Salad: A medley of seasonal fruits like berries, melon, kiwi, and citrus with a honey-lime drizzle.

Quinoa Salad: Quinoa, roasted vegetables, chickpeas, and a tahini-lemon dressing.

Salad Creations as a Lifestyle:

Salad creations are more than just a meal; they represent a lifestyle centered around fresh, nutritious, and delicious eating.

They encourage creativity in the kitchen and a mindful approach to food. Whether you're crafting a salad for a light lunch, a side dish, or a substantial dinner, the possibilities are limited only by your imagination. So, embrace the art of salad creation, and let your culinary talents shine as you compose beautiful and nourishing dishes that delight the senses and promote a healthy lifestyle.

Grilled Chicken Caesar Salad

The Grilled Chicken Caesar Salad is a classic that has stood the test of time for good reason. It's a dish that combines the crisp freshness of romaine lettuce, the savory richness of grilled chicken, the creaminess of Caesar dressing, and the zing of Parmesan cheese. This harmonious blend of flavors and textures makes it a go-to choose for salad lovers and a staple on restaurant menus. Let's dive into what makes the Grilled Chicken Caesar Salad so special and how to create a mouthwatering version at home.

The Elements of a Grilled Chicken Caesar Salad:

Grilled Chicken: The star of the salad, tender grilled chicken breast or thigh adds a hearty protein element, making this salad a satisfying meal on its own.

Romaine Lettuce: Crisp and crunchy romaine lettuce serves as the base of the salad, providing a refreshing contrast to the other ingredients.

Caesar Dressing: The creamy Caesar dressing is a key player, infusing the salad with a rich, garlic-forward flavor. Traditional Caesar dressing contains ingredients like anchovies, garlic, mayonnaise, and Parmesan cheese.

Croutons: Toasted croutons or bread cubes provide a delightful crunch and soak up the dressing's flavors.

Parmesan Cheese: Shaved or grated Parmesan cheese adds a salty, nutty kick that enhances the overall taste of the salad.

Why We Love Grilled Chicken Caesar Salad:

Satisfying and Balanced: It's a well-rounded meal that offers a balance of protein, greens, and carbohydrates, making it both delicious and filling.

Timeless Flavor: The combination of creamy dressing, savory chicken, and umami-rich Parmesan cheese creates a flavor profile that's both classic and irresistible.

Customizable: You can easily tailor your Grilled Chicken Caesar Salad to your preferences, adjusting the amount of dressing, adding extra ingredients like cherry tomatoes or avocado, or even switching to a different protein source.

Quick and Easy: It's a relatively quick and straightforward salad to assemble, making it perfect for weeknight dinners or a satisfying workday lunch.

How to Make a Grilled Chicken Caesar Salad:

Here's a simple recipe to create your own Grilled Chicken Caesar Salad at home:

Ingredients:

For the salad:

2 boneless, skinless chicken breasts

2 hearts of romaine lettuce, chopped

1 cup croutons

1/2 cup shaved or grated Parmesan cheese

For the Caesar dressing (homemade or store-bought):

1/4 cup mayonnaise

2 tablespoons grated Parmesan cheese

2 tablespoons fresh lemon juice

1 tablespoon Dijon mustard

1 garlic clove, minced

Salt and black pepper to taste

Instructions:

Black pepper and salt are used to season the chicken breasts. Grill the chicken over medium-high heat for about 6-8 minutes per side or until fully cooked (165°F or 74°C internal temperature). After a few minutes of repose, cut them into strips.

In a large bowl, combine the chopped romaine lettuce, croutons, and sliced grilled chicken.

In a separate bowl, whisk together the ingredients for the Caesar dressing until smooth. Adjust the seasoning to your taste.

Drizzle the Caesar dressing over the salad and toss everything together to ensure even coating.

Sprinkle the shaved or grated Parmesan cheese over the top.

Serve your Grilled Chicken Caesar Salad immediately, garnished with extra croutons and Parmesan cheese if desired.

Customization:

Add extra vegetables like cherry tomatoes, avocado slices, or roasted red peppers for additional flavor and nutrients.

Use homemade croutons for a personalized touch. Simply toss cubed bread with olive oil and seasonings, then bake until crisp.

Substitute the grilled chicken with other proteins like shrimp, salmon, or tofu for a unique twist.

A Grilled Chicken Caesar Salad is a timeless classic that combines crisp greens, savory grilled chicken, creamy Caesar dressing, and Parmesan cheese into a delightful culinary experience. Whether you're enjoying it as a refreshing lunch, a satisfying dinner, or even as a starter at a fancy restaurant, this salad is sure to tantalize your taste buds and satisfy your cravings for a harmonious blend of flavors and textures.

Quinoa and Avocado Salad

Quinoa and avocado salad is a vibrant, nutrient-packed dish that brings together the earthy goodness of quinoa, the creamy richness of avocados, and an array of fresh vegetables and herbs. This salad is not only a feast for the eyes with its colorful ingredients but also a celebration of flavor and wholesome nutrition. Whether you're a health-conscious foodie or simply seeking a delicious and satisfying meal, this salad deserves a place on your plate.

Key Ingredients:

Quinoa: Quinoa is a high-protein grain that serves as the foundation of this salad. It's gluten-free and rich in essential amino acids, fiber, vitamins, and minerals.

Avocado: Creamy, buttery avocados provide healthy monounsaturated fats, fiber, and a luscious texture to the salad.

Fresh Vegetables: A medley of fresh vegetables such as bell peppers, cherry tomatoes, cucumbers, and red onions add a burst of color, flavor, and essential nutrients.

Herbs: Fresh herbs like cilantro or parsley infuse the salad with brightness and herbaceous notes.

Lemon or Lime: Citrus juice, either from lemons or limes, contributes acidity and a zesty kick.

Olive Oil: Extra-virgin olive oil not only adds richness but also provides healthy fats.

Seasonings: Salt, black pepper, and optional spices like cumin or paprika enhance the salad's flavor profile.

Why We Love Quinoa and Avocado Salad:

Nutrient Density: This salad is a nutritional powerhouse, packing in protein, healthy fats, vitamins, minerals, and dietary fiber.

Versatility: You can customize it by adding your favorite vegetables, herbs, or proteins (such as grilled chicken or tofu) to suit your taste.

Balanced Meal: Quinoa and avocado salad can be a standalone meal, offering a balance of carbohydrates, proteins, and healthy fats.

Texture Play: It boasts a delightful mix of textures, from the fluffy quinoa to the creamy avocados, crisp vegetables, and fresh herbs.

Quick and Easy: It's relatively simple to prepare and can be made ahead for a convenient, ready-to-eat meal.

How to Make Quinoa and Avocado Salad:

Here's a basic recipe to create your own Quinoa and Avocado Salad:

Ingredients:

For the salad:

1 cup quinoa

2 ripe avocados, diced

1 cup cherry tomatoes, halved

1 cucumber, diced

1 red bell pepper, diced

1/4 cup red onion, finely chopped

1/4 cup fresh cilantro or parsley, chopped

For the dressing:

2 tablespoons extra-virgin olive oil

Juice of 1 lemon or lime

Salt and black pepper to taste

Instructions:

Rinse the quinoa thoroughly in a fine-mesh strainer. In a saucepan, combine the quinoa with 2 cups of water and a pinch of salt. After bringing to a boil, lower the heat to a simmer, cover, and cook the quinoa for about fifteen minutes, or until it is tender and the water has been absorbed. Turn off the heat and let it to cool.

In a large bowl, combine the cooked and cooled quinoa, diced avocados, cherry tomatoes, cucumber, red bell pepper, red onion, and fresh cilantro or parsley.

In a small bowl, whisk together the extra-virgin olive oil and the lemon or lime juice. To taste, add salt and black pepper for seasoning.

Drizzle the dressing over the salad and gently toss everything together to coat the ingredients evenly.

Taste and adjust the seasoning or add more lemon/lime juice if desired.

Serve your Quinoa and Avocado Salad immediately as a refreshing meal or side dish.

Customization:

Add protein: Add some prawns, tofu or grilled chicken to up the protein content.

Extra veggies: Experiment with additional vegetables like corn, roasted sweet potatoes, or diced zucchini.

Nuts and seeds: For added crunch and nutrition, sprinkle toasted nuts (e.g., almonds or walnuts) or seeds (e.g., sunflower or pumpkin seeds) on top.

Spice it up: Customize the flavor with your favorite spices or seasonings, such as smoked paprika or cumin.

Quinoa and avocado salad are celebration of freshness, flavor, and nutrition that appeals to a wide range of palates. Whether enjoyed as a light lunch, a side dish at a barbecue, or a wholesome dinner, it's a versatile and satisfying salad that showcases the beauty and deliciousness of whole, natural ingredients. So, grab your ingredients and start creating your own bowl of quinoa and avocado salad today.

Low-Key Dinners

Low-key dinners are a culinary concept that prioritizes simplicity, ease of preparation, and comfort. These meals are not about elaborate recipes or extravagant ingredients; instead, they focus on wholesome, familiar foods that soothe the soul and bring a sense of ease to the dining experience. Whether you're looking for a quick weeknight meal, a cozy dinner for one, or a relaxed family gathering, low-key dinners are the answer.

The Essence of Low-Key Dinners:

Minimal Effort, Maximum Comfort: Low-key dinners are all about simplicity. They require minimal preparation and cooking time, allowing you to unwind and savor the meal without stress.

Family Favorites: These meals often consist of beloved family recipes, tried-and-true classics, or dishes that evoke a sense of nostalgia.

Quality Ingredients: While the recipes may be straightforward, the emphasis is on using high-quality ingredients to enhance flavor and enjoyment.

Versatility: Low-key dinners can be adapted to accommodate various dietary preferences, making them suitable for everyone at the table

Examples of Low-Key Dinners:

Spaghetti Aglio e Olio: A classic Italian dish featuring spaghetti tossed with garlic-infused olive oil, red pepper flakes, and fresh parsley. This spaghetti recipe is tasty but easy.

Grilled Cheese Sandwich: The ultimate comfort food, a grilled cheese sandwich combines gooey melted cheese between slices of toasted bread. Add a cup of tomato soup for the perfect pairing.

Baked Potatoes: Load up baked potatoes with toppings like butter, sour cream, chives, and grated cheese. They're customizable and filling.

Omelette: Whisk eggs, add your favorite fillings like cheese, vegetables, or ham, and cook into a fluffy omelet. Serve it with a side salad for balance.

Taco Night: Set up a taco bar with tortillas, seasoned ground meat or beans, and an array of toppings like lettuce, tomatoes, cheese, salsa, and guacamole.

Pasta Salad: Combine cooked pasta with a medley of vegetables, olives, cheese, and a zesty vinaigrette dressing. It's a versatile dish that can be served cold or at room temperature.

Why We Love Low-Key Dinners:

Stress-Free Cooking: These meals are quick and easy to prepare, making them perfect for busy weeknights or when you want a break from complex recipes.

Comfort and Nostalgia: Low-key dinners often evoke feelings of comfort and nostalgia, reminding us of cherished family meals or childhood favorites.

Balanced Simplicity: They strike a balance between simplicity and flavor, allowing the ingredients to shine without unnecessary fuss.

Accessibility: The ingredients for low-key dinners are typically readily available, making them accessible to most home cooks.

Creating Your Own Low-Key Dinners:

The beauty of low-key dinners lies in their flexibility. You can personalize these meals to suit your taste and dietary preferences. Here are some tips for creating your own low-key dinners:

Start with a Base: Begin with a simple base like pasta, rice, potatoes, or bread. These ingredients provide substance and comfort.

Add Proteins: Incorporate proteins like eggs, beans, cheese, or grilled chicken to make the meal more substantial.

Season with Care: Use herbs, spices, and condiments to enhance flavor. Even a sprinkle of fresh herbs or a dash of hot sauce can elevate a dish.

Don't Forget Vegetables: Include vegetables, whether they're a side salad, roasted vegetables, or sautéed greens, to add freshness and nutrition.

Keep It Balanced: Aim for a balanced plate with a mix of carbohydrates, proteins, and vegetables for a well-rounded meal.

Embrace Leftovers: Low-key dinners are excellent for using up leftovers from previous meals, reducing food waste.

Low-key dinners are a celebration of simplicity, comfort, and the joy of savoring uncomplicated yet delicious food. Whether you're sharing a meal with loved ones or indulging in a peaceful solo dinner, these dishes bring a sense of ease and contentment to the table. So, next time you're in need of a stress-free meal that warms the heart and satisfies the palate, consider whipping up a low-key dinner that speaks to your soul.

Baked Salmon with Dill Sauce

Baked salmon with dill sauce is a culinary masterpiece that combines the rich, buttery texture of salmon with the bright and refreshing flavors of dill and lemon. This dish is not only a delight for the taste buds but also a celebration of nutritious and heart-healthy eating. Whether you're looking for a special meal for a gathering or a satisfying weeknight dinner, baked salmon with dill sauce is a surefire winner that leaves a lasting impression.

Key Ingredients:

Salmon: The star of the show, salmon is fatty fish rich in omega-3 fatty acids, which are known for their heart-healthy benefits. It's a protein-packed foundation for this dish.

Fresh Dill: Fragrant and herbaceous, fresh dill provides a burst of flavor that complements the salmon beautifully.

Lemon: The citrusy tang of lemon juice and zest adds brightness and zing to the dish.

Greek Yogurt or Sour Cream: Creamy Greek yogurt or sour cream forms the base of the dill sauce, lending a luscious texture and tangy flavor.

Dijon Mustard: A touch of Dijon mustard gives the sauce a subtle kick and enhances its depth of flavor.

Garlic: Minced garlic infuses the sauce with a gentle but aromatic essence.

Salt and Pepper: To season the salmon and the sauce, bringing all the flavors together.

Why We Love Baked Salmon with Dill Sauce:

Health Benefits: Salmon is packed with omega-3 fatty acids, which have been associated with reduced risk of heart disease and improved brain health.

Flavor Harmony: The combination of rich salmon, zesty lemon, aromatic dill, and creamy sauce creates a harmonious balance of flavors.

Quick and Easy: Baking salmon is a fuss-free cooking method, making this dish accessible even to home cooks with minimal experience.

Elegant Presentation: Baked salmon with dill sauce is visually appealing, making it an excellent choice for special occasions or when you want to impress guests.

How to Prepare Dill Sauce for Baked Salmon:

Here's a simple recipe to create your own Baked Salmon with Dill Sauce:

Ingredients:

For the salmon:

4 salmon fillets (6-8 ounces each)

Olive oil for brushing

Salt and black pepper to taste

Lemon slices for garnish (optional)

For the dill sauce:

1/2 cup Greek yogurt or sour cream

2 tablespoons fresh dill, chopped

1 tablespoon lemon juice

1 teaspoon lemon zest

1 teaspoon Dijon mustard

1 garlic clove, minced

Salt and black pepper to taste

Instructions:

Preheat your oven to 375°F (190°C). Grease a baking sheet gently or line it with parchment paper.

After the baking sheet is ready, put the salmon fillets on it. Brush each fillet with olive oil and season with salt and black pepper.

Bake the salmon in the preheated oven for approximately 12-15 minutes, or until the salmon easily flakes with a fork. Depending on the thickness of the fillets, cooking times can change.

Make the dill sauce while the fish bakes. In a small bowl, combine the Greek yogurt or sour cream, fresh dill, lemon juice, lemon zest, Dijon mustard, minced garlic, salt, and black pepper. Mix until well combined.

After the salmon is cooked, take it out of the oven and give it some time to rest.

Serve the baked salmon on individual plates, drizzled with the dill sauce. If preferred, garnish with more dill and lemon slices.

Customization:

For a crispy crust, you can broil the salmon for a minute or two after baking.

Add a pinch of cayenne pepper to the dill sauce for a subtle spicy kick.

Pair your baked salmon with a side of steamed asparagus, roasted potatoes, or a fresh green salad for a complete meal.

Baked salmon with dill sauce is a true culinary masterpiece that combines the heart-healthy benefits of salmon with the vibrant and refreshing flavors of dill and lemon. It's a dish that's not only delicious but also impressively nutritious, making it an ideal choice for health-conscious foodies and those seeking a memorable dining experience. Whether you're hosting a special dinner or treating yourself to a comforting meal, this dish delivers a symphony of flavors and a sense of wholesome indulgence.

Turkey and Sweet Potato Casserole

Turkey and sweet potato casserole is a comforting and satisfying dish that brings together the savory goodness of roasted turkey, the natural sweetness of sweet potatoes, and a medley of flavors and textures. This casserole is a perfect choice for a hearty family dinner, a festive holiday feast, or any occasion when you crave the warm embrace of home-cooked comfort food.

Key Ingredients:

Turkey: Roasted or shredded turkey provides a substantial source of lean protein and a rich, savory flavor.

Sweet Potatoes: Sweet potatoes are the star of the dish, adding natural sweetness, creaminess, and essential nutrients like beta-carotene.

Vegetables: A mix of sautéed onions, garlic, and other vegetables such as bell peppers, corn, or peas can enhance the flavor and provide color and nutrition.

Herbs and Seasonings: A blend of herbs like thyme, sage, or rosemary, along with salt, pepper, and optional spices, adds depth and aroma to the casserole.

Creamy Sauce: A velvety sauce made with ingredients like chicken broth, heavy cream, or a dairy-free alternative helps bind the casserole and infuse it with richness.

Toppings: Crispy toppings like breadcrumbs, grated cheese, or crispy fried onions add texture and a layer of indulgence

Why We Love Turkey and Sweet Potato Casserole:

Comforting and Wholesome: It's a comforting and hearty meal that evokes a sense of homey warmth and nostalgia.

Perfect for Leftovers: If you have leftover turkey from a holiday meal, this casserole is an excellent way to repurpose it into a delicious dish.

Balanced Nutrition: The combination of turkey and sweet potatoes provides a balance of protein, complex carbohydrates, and vitamins, making it a nutritious choice.

Versatility: You can customize the casserole by adding your favorite vegetables, herbs, or seasonings to suit your taste.

How to Prepare Sweet Potato and Turkey Casserole:

Here's a basic recipe to create your own Turkey and Sweet Potato Casserole:

Ingredients:

2 cups cooked turkey, shredded or diced

3 large sweet potatoes, peeled and cubed

1 onion, chopped

2 cloves garlic, minced

1 cup mixed vegetables (e.g., corn, peas, bell peppers)

1/2 cup chicken broth

1/2 cup heavy cream or a substitute made without dairy

2 tablespoons butter or olive oil

1 teaspoon dried thyme

Salt and black pepper to taste

Optional toppings: breadcrumbs, grated cheese, or crispy fried onions

Instructions:

Preheat your oven to 350°F (175°C) and grease a casserole dish.

Place the sweet potato cubes in a pot of boiling water and cook until they are tender, about 10-15 minutes. Drain and set aside.

Melt the butter or olive oil in a big skillet over medium heat. After adding the chopped onion, simmer it for three to five minutes, or until it turns transparent. Add the minced garlic and continue cooking for one more minute.

Stir in the cooked turkey, mixed vegetables, thyme, salt, and black pepper. The vegetables should be sautéed for a few minutes to make them soft.

In a separate saucepan, combine the chicken broth and heavy cream (or dairy-free alternative) and heat over low heat until warmed.

Place the cooked sweet potato cubes in a large mixing bowl. Pour the chicken broth and cream mixture over the sweet potatoes and mash them until smooth. You can use a potato masher or an electric mixer for this step.

In the prepared casserole dish, spread a layer of the mashed sweet potatoes. Top it with the turkey and vegetable mixture.

Add another layer of the mashed sweet potatoes on top, spreading it evenly.

If desired, sprinkle the casserole with your choice of toppings, such as breadcrumbs, grated cheese, or crispy fried onions.

Bake for 25 to 30 minutes, or until the casserole is heated through and the top is golden brown, in a preheated oven.

Before serving, allow it to cool for a few minutes.

Customization:

Experiment with different vegetables, herbs, or seasonings to create your own flavor profile.

For a healthier twist, use a dairy-free cream substitute and whole-grain breadcrumbs.

Add a sprinkle of grated Parmesan or cheddar cheese for extra flavor.

Turkey and sweet potato casserole are a heartwarming dish that combines the wholesome goodness of sweet potatoes with the savory richness of turkey, creating a symphony of flavors and textures that evoke the comforts of home. Whether you're enjoying it as a family dinner, a holiday favorite, or a creative way to use up leftover turkey, this casserole is sure to warm your heart and satisfy your appetite with its hearty and delicious appeal.

Chapter 4

Snacks and Sides for Gentle Grazing

Snacking and enjoying sides throughout the day can be a delightful way to keep your energy levels steady and satisfy your taste buds without the commitment of a full meal. When it comes to gentle grazing, the focus is on nourishing your body with wholesome, balanced, and flavorful options. Whether you're looking for a mid-morning pick-me-up, an afternoon snack, or a little something to accompany your main course, here are some enticing snacks and sides to elevate your grazing experience.

Nuts and Seeds:

Trail Mix: Create your own blend of nuts, seeds, and dried fruits for a customizable and nutrient-packed snack.

Almonds: A handful of almonds offers a satisfying crunch and a dose of healthy fats, fiber, and protein.

Chia Pudding: Mix chia seeds with almond milk, honey, and a dash of vanilla for a creamy and nutritious pudding.

Fresh Fruits:

Apple Slices with Peanut Butter: The classic combination of crisp apple slices and creamy peanut butter is a timeless favorite.

Berries and Greek Yogurt: Top a bowl of Greek yogurt with fresh berries for a protein-rich and antioxidant-packed snack.

Citrus Salad: A medley of citrus fruits drizzled with honey and a sprinkle of mint leaves is a refreshing and vitamin C-rich choice.

Vegetable Delights:

Hummus and Veggie Sticks: Dip cucumber, carrot, and bell pepper sticks into hummus for a satisfying and nutritious snack.

Guacamole with Whole Grain Chips: Creamy guacamole pairs perfectly with whole-grain tortilla chips for a dose of healthy fats and fiber.

Crispy Kale Chips: Baked kale chips seasoned with olive oil, salt, and your favorite spices are a crunchy and guilt-free snack.

Dairy and Dairy Alternatives:

Cheese and Whole Grain Crackers: Enjoy a variety of cheeses with whole grain crackers for a satisfying combination of flavors and textures.

Yogurt Parfait: Layer yogurt with granola and fresh fruit to create a parfait that's both creamy and crunchy.

Cottage Cheese and Pineapple: A scoop of cottage cheese paired with pineapple chunks is a protein-rich and sweet-savory option.

Homemade Snacks:

Energy Bites: Make your own energy bites with oats, honey, nut butter, and add-ins like chocolate chips or dried fruit.

Popcorn: Air-popped popcorn with a sprinkle of nutritional yeast or your favorite seasoning blend is a guilt-free and whole-grain snack.

Baked Sweet Potato Fries: Slice sweet potatoes into fries, season with your preferred spices, and bake until crispy for a tasty and nutritious side.

International Flavors:

Sushi Rolls: Savor bite-sized sushi rolls filled with fresh vegetables, fish, or avocado for a unique and savory snack.

Greek Tzatziki: Enjoy Greek yogurt-based tzatziki with pita bread or cucumber slices for a tangy and refreshing dip.

Samosas: These savory pastries filled with spiced vegetables or meat are a delightful option for a savory snack.

Sweet Treats:

Dark Chocolate: A square of high-quality dark chocolate can satisfy your sweet tooth and provide antioxidants.

Fruit Sorbet: Savor a scoop of fruit sorbet for a refreshing and naturally sweet dessert.

Banana Ice Cream: Blend frozen bananas until creamy for a dairy-free and guilt-free ice cream alternative.

Gentle grazing with snacks and sides offers a variety of flavors, textures, and nutrients to keep you fueled and satisfied throughout the day. Whether you prefer something sweet, savory, or a combination of both, these options provide a delicious and nourishing way to curb hunger and indulge your taste buds without the need for a full meal. So, embrace the art of gentle grazing, and discover the joy of savoring these wholesome bites between your main courses.

Nutrient-Packed Snacks

Nutrient-packed snacks are more than just delicious treats; they're small but mighty powerhouses that provide your body with essential vitamins, minerals, fiber, and energy to keep you going throughout the day. These snacks offer a balanced combination of macronutrients (carbohydrates, proteins, and fats) and micronutrients (vitamins and minerals), making them a smart choice for maintaining good health and satisfying your hunger. Whether you're looking for a quick pick-me-up between meals or a tasty way to refuel after a workout, nutrient-packed snacks have you covered.

Why Nutrient-Packed Snacks Matter:

Sustained Energy: Snacks that contain a balance of carbohydrates, proteins, and healthy fats provide you with a steady release of energy, helping you stay alert and focused.

Improved Nutrient Intake: These snacks are a convenient way to fill nutritional gaps in your diet, ensuring you get the vitamins and minerals your body needs.

Appetite Control: Nutrient-dense snacks can help control your appetite and prevent overeating during main meals.

Support for Active Lifestyles: Athletes and active individuals can benefit from nutrient-packed snacks that aid in muscle recovery and provide sustained energy during workouts.

Nutrient-Packed Snack Ideas:

Greek Yogurt with Berries: Greek yogurt is rich in protein, while berries provide antioxidants and fiber. Add a drizzle of honey and a sprinkle of nuts for extra flavor and nutrients.

Hummus and Veggie Sticks: Hummus offers plant-based protein and healthy fats, while colorful vegetable sticks provide vitamins and fiber.

Almonds or Mixed Nuts: A small handful of nuts delivers healthy fats, protein, and a variety of vitamins and minerals. Opt for unsalted or lightly salted varieties.

Hard-Boiled Eggs: Eggs are a fantastic source of protein and nutrients like choline. For added taste, season them with a little salt and pepper.

Whole Grain Crackers with Nut Butter: Whole grain crackers offer fiber and complex carbohydrates, while nut butter adds healthy fats and protein.

Trail Mix: Create your own trail mix with a mix of nuts, seeds, dried fruits, and a touch of dark chocolate for a satisfying sweet-savory blend.

Oatmeal with Nut Butter: A small bowl of oatmeal with a dollop of nut butter and a drizzle of honey is a warm and satisfying snack.

Cottage Cheese and Fruit: Cottage cheese is packed with protein and pairs beautifully with fresh or canned fruits for a creamy and sweet snack.

Avocado Toast: Top whole grain toast with sliced avocado and a sprinkle of salt, pepper, and chili flakes for a nutrient-rich snack.

Cucumber Slices with Tuna: Scoop canned tuna onto cucumber slices for a low-carb, high-protein snack.

Smoothie: Blend your favorite fruits with Greek yogurt or plant-based protein powder for a refreshing and nutrient-packed beverage.

Edamame: These young soybeans are loaded with protein and make for a satisfying and crunchy snack.

Chia Pudding: Mix chia seeds with almond milk, honey, and your choice of toppings like fresh fruit or nuts for a creamy and nutrient-dense pudding.

Yogurt Parfait: Layer yogurt with granola and fresh berries for a balance of protein, fiber, and antioxidants.

Roasted Chickpeas: Seasoned and roasted chickpeas are a crunchy and protein-packed snack with a delightful flavor kick.

Customizing Your Snacks:

Feel free to customize your nutrient-packed snacks to suit your preferences and dietary needs. You can adjust portion sizes, experiment with different flavors, and choose organic or local ingredients when available. Remember that variety is key to ensuring you get a wide range of nutrients, so don't be afraid to mix and match your favorite options.

Nutrient-packed snacks are a delicious and convenient way to support your overall health and well-being. By choosing these snacks, you're not only satisfying your cravings but also nourishing your body with the essential nutrients it needs to thrive. So, the next time you reach for a snack, consider the wholesome goodness of nutrient-packed options and enjoy the benefits of balanced and satisfying snacking.

Greek Yogurt with Honey and Berries

Greek yogurt with honey and berries is a simple yet divine combination that brings together creamy yogurt, the natural sweetness of honey, and the burst of flavors from fresh or frozen berries. This delightful treat is not only a feast for the taste buds but also a nutritional powerhouse that's perfect for breakfast, a snack, or even a light dessert. Let's delve into why this combination is so beloved and how to savor it to the fullest.

Key Ingredients:

Greek Yogurt: Greek yogurt is thicker and creamier than regular yogurt due to the straining process that removes excess whey. It's also rich in protein, probiotics, and calcium.

Honey: Honey adds a natural sweetness and a touch of floral flavor. It's not only delicious but also boasts antioxidants and potential health benefits.

Berries: Fresh berries like strawberries, blueberries, raspberries, or blackberries provide a juicy burst of flavor, vibrant color, and a host of vitamins, minerals, and antioxidants.

Why We Love Greek Yogurt with Honey and Berries:

Balanced Nutrition: This combination offers a balanced mix of protein from Greek yogurt, natural sugars from honey, and a range of nutrients from berries.

Creamy and Sweet: The creamy yogurt pairs beautifully with the sweet honey and the tartness of the berries, creating a harmonious blend of textures and flavors.

Versatility: Enjoy it as a breakfast parfait, a midday snack, or even a light dessert. It's a versatile treat that suits various occasions.

Quick and Easy: It takes mere minutes to prepare and requires minimal ingredients, making it a convenient choice for busy schedules.

How to Make Greek Yogurt with Honey and Berries:

Here's a simple recipe to create your own Greek Yogurt with Honey and Berries:

Ingredients:

1 cup Greek yogurt (plain or vanilla-flavored)

1-2 tablespoons honey (adjust to taste)

1 cup fresh or frozen mixed berries (strawberries, blueberries, raspberries, blackberries)

Optional toppings: granola, chopped nuts, or a sprinkle of cinnamon

Instructions:

Prepare the Berries:

If using fresh berries, rinse and drain them. You can also slice larger berries like strawberries.

If using frozen berries, thaw them in the refrigerator or microwave them briefly until they reach your desired temperature.

Layer the Yogurt and Berries:

Start with a layer of Greek yogurt at the bottom of a serving bowl or glass.

Add a spoonful of honey over the yogurt, drizzling it evenly.

Place a portion of your berries on top of the yogurt and honey.

Repeat the Layers:

Continue layering yogurt, honey, and berries until you've used up your ingredients.

Add Toppings (Optional):

If desired, top your Greek yogurt with granola for a delightful crunch, chopped nuts for extra texture, or a sprinkle of cinnamon for warmth and flavor.

Serve and Enjoy:

Serve your Greek Yogurt with Honey and Berries immediately and savor each spoonful of this delicious and wholesome treat.

Customization:

Customize the sweetness by adjusting the amount of honey to suit your taste.

Experiment with different berries or a mix of berries to create your ideal flavor combination.

Enhance the texture with various toppings, such as chia seeds, coconut flakes, or a dollop of almond butter.

Greek yogurt with honey and berries is a delectable and nutrient-packed treat that strikes a harmonious balance between creamy, sweet, and tart. Whether you enjoy it for breakfast to kickstart your day, as a refreshing snack in the afternoon, or as a guilt-free dessert after dinner, this combination never fails to satisfy your cravings and nourish your body. So, treat yourself to this wholesome delight and relish the goodness of each spoonful.

Rice Cakes with Hummus

Rice cakes with hummus make for a delightful and wholesome snack that marries the crispiness of rice cakes with the creamy richness of hummus. This simple yet satisfying combination offers a perfect blend of textures and flavors that can be enjoyed as a quick midday pick-me-up, a pre-workout snack, or a light appetizer. Let's explore why this pairing is so beloved and how to savor it to the fullest.

Key Ingredients:

Rice Cakes: Rice cakes are low in calories and provide a satisfying crunch. They serve as a blank canvas for various toppings.

Hummus: Hummus is a creamy spread made from chickpeas, tahini, olive oil, lemon juice, garlic, and seasonings. It's a good source of plant-based protein, healthy fats, and fiber.

Why We Love Rice Cakes with Hummus:

Textural Harmony: The crispy rice cakes contrast beautifully with the velvety, creamy hummus, creating a delightful mouthfeel.

Balanced Nutrition: This snack offers a balance of carbohydrates from the rice cakes and protein and healthy fats from the hummus, making it satisfying and energizing.

Quick and Easy: It's a no-fuss snack that requires minimal preparation and can be assembled in a matter of minutes.

Versatility: You can customize your rice cakes with hummus by adding various toppings or seasonings to suit your taste.

How to Make Rice Cakes with Hummus:

Creating your own Rice Cakes with Hummus is as easy as it gets. Here's a basic guide to making this delicious snack:

Ingredients:

Rice cakes (choose your preferred flavor or type)

Hummus (store-bought or homemade)

Optional toppings: sliced cucumbers, cherry tomatoes, baby carrots, olives, fresh herbs, or a drizzle of olive oil

Instructions:

Prepare the Rice Cakes:

Lay out the desired number of rice cakes on a clean surface.

Spread Hummus:

Using a butter knife or a small spoon, spread a generous layer of hummus onto each rice cake.

Add Toppings (Optional):

Get creative with your toppings! Arrange thin slices of cucumber, halved cherry tomatoes, baby carrots, pitted olives, or fresh herbs like parsley or basil on top of the hummus.

Drizzle with Olive Oil (Optional):

For an extra touch of flavor, drizzle a small amount of olive oil over your rice cakes with hummus.

Serve and Enjoy:

Arrange your rice cakes with hummus on a plate, and enjoy this satisfying, crunchy, and creamy snack.

Customization:

Spice it up: Sprinkle a pinch of paprika, cayenne pepper, or za'atar on top of the hummus for a flavor kick.

Fresh and zesty: Squeeze a bit of lemon juice over the hummus for a zesty twist.

Protein boost: Add a few slices of roasted red pepper or grilled chicken for extra protein.

Vegan delight: Opt for a dairy-free hummus to keep this snack vegan-friendly.

Rice cakes with hummus offer a delightful contrast of textures and a harmonious blend of flavors that are sure to satisfy your cravings and keep you fueled throughout the day. Whether you're enjoying them as a solo snack or sharing them with friends and family, this pairing is a testament to the joy of simplicity and deliciousness in snacking. So, embrace the crispy and creamy goodness of rice cakes with hummus and indulge in this nutritious and tasty treat.

Satisfying Sides

Satisfying sides are the unsung heroes of any meal, transforming a simple dish into a well-rounded and memorable culinary experience. These delectable companions bring an array of flavors, textures, and nutritional benefits to the table, enhancing the overall enjoyment of your main course. Whether you're aiming to add a burst of color, a touch of indulgence, or a dose of wholesome goodness to your plate, satisfying sides are here to elevate your meals.

The Magic of Satisfying Sides:

Complementing Flavors: Sides are designed to complement the flavors of the main dish, offering a harmonious contrast or enhancement.

Texture Variety: They introduce a variety of textures, from crispy and crunchy to creamy and velvety, providing a sensory delight.

Nutritional Boost: Sides often contribute essential nutrients, such as fiber, vitamins, and minerals, enriching the nutritional profile of your meal.

Creative Expression: Sides are a canvas for creativity, allowing you to experiment with flavors, ingredients, and cooking techniques.

Versatile Satisfying Sides:

Vegetable Medleys: Sautéed, roasted, or steamed vegetables like broccoli, carrots, and bell peppers provide a colorful and nutritious addition to any plate.

Mashed Potatoes: Creamy and buttery mashed potatoes are a classic side that pairs perfectly with roasted meats and gravy.

Garlic Bread: Warm, crusty garlic bread is a beloved side, ideal for dipping into soups or enjoying with pasta.

Coleslaw: A tangy coleslaw made from shredded cabbage and a zesty dressing adds a refreshing crunch to BBQs and sandwiches.

Rice Pilaf: Fragrant rice pilaf, cooked with herbs and vegetables, brings a touch of elegance to any meal.

Quinoa Salad: Quinoa salads, tossed with fresh vegetables and a vinaigrette, offer a protein-rich and gluten-free option.

Cornbread: Sweet and savory cornbread is a Southern favorite that pairs wonderfully with chili and stews.

Creamed Spinach: Creamed spinach is a luxurious side that beautifully complements grilled meats and fish.

Fruit Salsas: Fresh fruit salsas, made with ingredients like mango, pineapple, or peach, bring a burst of sweetness to grilled chicken or fish.

Avocado Fries: Avocado fries, coated in crispy breadcrumbs, offer a unique twist on traditional French fries.

Couscous with Dried Fruits: Couscous paired with dried fruits and nuts provides a delightful blend of textures and flavors.

Stuffed Mushrooms: Stuffed mushrooms filled with cheese, herbs, and breadcrumbs are a flavorful appetizer or side.

Roasted Root Vegetables: Roasted root vegetables like sweet potatoes, parsnips, and turnips are hearty and satisfying.

Customizing Your Sides:

Feel free to customize your satisfying sides to suit your preferences and dietary needs. You can adjust seasonings, incorporate regional flavors, or opt for healthier cooking methods like grilling or air frying. The key is to experiment and find what complements your main dish and satisfies your palate.

Satisfying sides are the unsung heroes that elevate your meals from ordinary to extraordinary. They not only enhance the overall dining experience but also provide a wonderful opportunity for culinary creativity and self-expression. So, embrace the world of satisfying sides, and let your taste buds embark on a delightful journey of flavors and textures with each bite.

Mashed Potatoes with Garlic and Herbs

Mashed potatoes with garlic and herbs is a beloved side dish that takes the comforting creaminess of mashed potatoes and elevates it with the aromatic richness of garlic and the earthy flavors of fresh herbs. This classic comfort food is a perfect accompaniment to a wide range of main courses and is often associated with holiday feasts and family gatherings. Let's dive into the details of why mashed potatoes with garlic and herbs are so adored and how to prepare this delectable dish.

Key Ingredients:

Potatoes: Russet potatoes or Yukon Gold potatoes are commonly used for mashed potatoes due to their starchy and creamy texture.

Garlic: Fresh garlic cloves add a pungent and savory flavor to the dish when roasted or sautéed.

Herbs: Fresh herbs like rosemary, thyme, or chives bring a burst of aromatic freshness to the mashed potatoes.

Dairy: Butter, cream, or milk is used to achieve the creamy consistency and add a rich, velvety flavor.

Seasonings: Salt and pepper are essential for enhancing the taste of the mashed potatoes.

Why We Love Mashed Potatoes with Garlic and Herbs:
Aromatic Complexity: Garlic and fresh herbs introduce a depth of flavor and fragrance that transforms plain mashed potatoes into something extraordinary.

Comforting Creaminess: The creamy and fluffy texture of mashed potatoes provides a comforting and satisfying experience.

Versatile Pairing: This side dish pairs seamlessly with a variety of main courses, from roast chicken to grilled steak or vegetarian options.

Holiday Tradition: Mashed potatoes with garlic and herbs are often a cherished part of holiday feasts and special occasions, bringing a sense of nostalgia and togetherness.

How to Make Mashed Potatoes with Garlic and Herbs:

Here's a basic recipe to create your own Mashed Potatoes with Garlic and Herbs:

Ingredients:

4 large russet or Yukon Gold potatoes, peeled and cut into chunks

4-6 garlic cloves, peeled and minced or left whole for roasting

1/2 cup unsalted butter, at room temperature

1/2 cup milk or heavy cream

2 tablespoons fresh herbs (e.g., rosemary, thyme, or chives), finely chopped

Salt and black pepper, to taste

Instructions:

Boil the Potatoes:

Place the potato chunks in a large pot of salted water and bring to a boil. Cook until the potatoes are fork-tender, about 15-20 minutes.

Roast or Sauté the Garlic (Optional):

If you prefer a milder garlic flavor, sauté the minced garlic in a small amount of butter or olive oil until fragrant but not browned. Alternatively, roast whole garlic cloves in the oven until they become soft and golden.

Drain and Mash:

Drain the cooked potatoes and return them to the pot. Mash the potatoes using a potato masher or a potato ricer until smooth and free of lumps.

Add Butter and Milk/Cream:

Incorporate the butter and milk or cream into the mashed potatoes, stirring until the butter is fully melted and the mixture is creamy.

Add Garlic and Herbs:

Fold in the roasted or sautéed garlic and fresh herbs, ensuring they are evenly distributed throughout the mashed potatoes.

Season to Taste:

Season with salt and black pepper to your liking. Taste and adjust as needed.

Serve Hot:

Transfer the mashed potatoes with garlic and herbs to a serving dish and serve hot.

Customization:

For extra creaminess, you can use heavy cream instead of milk.

Feel free to mix and match your favorite herbs or add a sprinkle of grated Parmesan cheese for an extra layer of flavor.

If you prefer a rustic texture, leave the skins on the potatoes for added fiber and nutrients.

Mashed potatoes with garlic and herbs are the epitome of comfort food, offering a harmonious blend of creamy texture and savory flavors. Whether you're enjoying them on a special occasion or as a comforting side to your weeknight dinner, these mashed potatoes are sure to bring a smile to your face and warmth to your heart. So, indulge in this timeless classic and savor the delightful marriage of garlic, herbs, and velvety potatoes with each heavenly spoonful.

Steamed Asparagus with Lemon Butter

Steamed asparagus with lemon butter is a delightful side dish that combines the earthy, tender-crisp crunch of asparagus with the zesty brightness of lemon-infused butter. This elegant and easy-to-prepare dish is not only visually appealing but also a perfect complement to a wide range of main courses, from grilled salmon to roasted chicken or vegetarian entrees. Let's explore why steamed asparagus with lemon butter is so beloved and how to prepare it to perfection.

Key Ingredients:

Asparagus: Fresh, vibrant-green asparagus spears are the star of this dish. Look for spears that are firm, with tightly closed tips and minimal browning.

Butter: Unsalted butter forms the base of the lemon-infused sauce, providing richness and a luscious mouthfeel.

Lemon: Fresh lemon juice and zest infuse the dish with a tangy and citrusy flavor, elevating the asparagus to a whole new level.

Salt and Pepper: These seasonings are essential for enhancing the taste of the asparagus and balancing the flavors.

Why We Love Steamed Asparagus with Lemon Butter:
Vibrant Flavors: The combination of asparagus, lemon, and butter creates a symphony of flavors that are both bright and indulgent.

Versatile Pairing: This side dish pairs beautifully with a wide range of proteins, making it suitable for various meals and occasions.

Quick Preparation: With minimal ingredients and straightforward cooking methods, steamed asparagus with lemon butter is a breeze to make.

Health Benefits: Asparagus is a nutrient powerhouse, packed with vitamins, minerals, and fiber, making this side dish not only delicious but also nutritious.

How to Make Steamed Asparagus with Lemon Butter:

Here's a basic recipe to create your own Steamed Asparagus with

Lemon Butter:

Ingredients:

1 bunch of fresh asparagus spears (about 1 pound)

4 tablespoons unsalted butter

Zest and juice of one lemon

Salt and black pepper, to taste

Lemon wedges or slices (for garnish, optional)

Instructions:

Prepare the Asparagus:

Wash the asparagus under cold running water and trim off the tough ends by snapping them off at their natural breaking point. You can also use a knife to trim them.

Steam the Asparagus:

Fill a large pot with a few inches of water and bring it to a boil. Place a steamer basket or a heatproof colander over the pot.

Arrange the trimmed asparagus in a single layer in the steamer basket.

Cover the pot and steam the asparagus for about 3-5 minutes, or until they are tender-crisp. The cooking time may vary depending on the thickness of the asparagus.

Prepare the Lemon Butter Sauce:

While the asparagus is steaming, melt the butter in a small saucepan over low heat. Add the lemon zest and juice, stirring to combine. Season with a pinch of salt and black pepper. Keep the sauce warm over low heat.

Serve the Dish:

Transfer the steamed asparagus to a serving platter or individual plates. Drizzle the lemon butter sauce over the asparagus.

Garnish with lemon wedges or slices, if desired, for an extra touch of citrus freshness.

Enjoy:

Serve the steamed asparagus with lemon butter immediately, savoring the vibrant flavors and contrasting textures.

Customization:

Add a sprinkle of freshly grated Parmesan cheese or toasted almonds for additional flavor and texture.

Experiment with other fresh herbs like chopped parsley, dill, or chives to enhance the dish's aroma and visual appeal.

For a lighter version, use olive oil instead of butter, creating a lemon vinaigrette with the lemon juice and zest.

Steamed asparagus with lemon butter is a testament to the beauty of simplicity in cooking. It's a side dish that celebrates the natural flavors of asparagus while enhancing them with the bright and zesty notes of lemon-infused butter. Whether you're

serving it as part of a holiday feast or as a weeknight accompaniment to your favorite protein, this dish is sure to bring a touch of elegance and refreshment to your table. So, embrace the pairing of asparagus and lemon, and let your taste buds revel in the deliciousness of this bright and vibrant side dish.

Chapter 5

Desserts that Won't Upset Your Stomach

Desserts are a sweet and satisfying way to end a meal or indulge in a delightful treat. However, for some individuals with sensitive stomachs or dietary restrictions, certain desserts can lead to discomfort or digestive issues. The good news is that there are plenty of dessert options that can satisfy your sweet tooth without causing digestive upset. These desserts prioritize ingredients and preparation methods that are gentle on the stomach, making them ideal for those seeking a more stomach-friendly indulgence.

1. **Fruit Salad:**

Fresh fruit salads are light, refreshing, and easy to digest. They provide natural sweetness and are packed with vitamins, fiber, and antioxidants.

2. **Banana Ice Cream:**

Blend frozen ripe bananas into a creamy, dairy-free ice cream. It's a guilt-free and soothing dessert option.

3. Oatmeal Cookies:

Homemade oatmeal cookies made with whole-grain oats and natural sweeteners like honey or mashed bananas can be easier on the stomach than traditional cookies.

4. Rice Pudding:

Creamy rice pudding made with rice, milk, and a touch of vanilla and cinnamon can be a comforting, mild dessert.

5. Yogurt Parfait:

Layer yogurt with fresh berries and a sprinkle of granola for a delightful combination of creaminess, sweetness, and crunch.

6. Baked Apples:

Baked apples with a touch of cinnamon and a drizzle of honey provide natural sweetness and are easy to digest.

7. Chia Seed Pudding:

Chia seeds soaked in almond milk or yogurt create a pudding-like dessert that's gentle on the stomach and high in fiber.

8. Mashed Sweet Potatoes:

Mashed sweet potatoes with a sprinkle of cinnamon and a dollop of Greek yogurt are not only tasty but also soothing.

9. Ginger Cookies:

Ginger has been known to help with digestion. Homemade ginger cookies can provide a sweet and stomach-soothing option.

10. Coconut Rice Cakes:

Top rice cakes with a thin layer of coconut yogurt and fresh fruit for a light and flavorful dessert.

11. Sorbet:

Sorbet made from real fruit puree is dairy-free and offers a refreshing and gentle dessert option.

12. Smoothie Bowls:

Blend your favorite fruits and yogurt or almond milk into a creamy smoothie bowl, topped with nuts, seeds, and fresh berries.

13. Angel Food Cake:

Angel food cake is lighter and less rich than many other cakes, making it easier on the stomach.

14. Dark Chocolate:

Dark chocolate with a high cocoa content contains less sugar and dairy, which can be easier to digest for some people.

15. Popsicles:

Homemade fruit popsicles made from pureed fruit and water are a fun and soothing way to enjoy dessert.

16. Almond Butter and Banana Bites:

Spread almond butter on banana slices and add a drizzle of honey for a quick and nutritious dessert.

17. Avocado Chocolate Mousse:

Avocado-based chocolate mousse is creamy, dairy-free, and full of healthy fats.

When enjoying desserts that won't upset your stomach, it's essential to pay attention to portion sizes and listen to your body's signals. While these dessert options are generally gentle on the stomach, individual tolerance may vary. Additionally, it's a good idea to consult with a healthcare professional if you have specific dietary concerns or food sensitivities to ensure you're making the best choices for your stomach health.

Fruit-Based Delights

Fruit-based delights are a delectable and wholesome category of desserts that celebrate the natural sweetness and vibrant flavors of fresh fruits. These desserts prioritize the use of fruits as the star ingredient, allowing their natural sugars, colors, and textures to shine. Whether you're craving something light and refreshing or indulging in a sweet treat that aligns with your health-conscious lifestyle, fruit-based delights offer a delightful and nutritious option.

Why We Love Fruit-Based Delights:

Natural Sweetness: Fruits are naturally sweet, making them the perfect foundation for delicious desserts without the need for excessive added sugars.

Vibrant Colors: The wide array of colors in fruits not only adds visual appeal but also signifies an abundance of vitamins, minerals, and antioxidants.

Balanced Nutrition: Fruits provide essential nutrients, including dietary fiber, vitamins, and minerals, making fruit-based desserts both tasty and nutritious.

Variety: There is an endless variety of fruits available, allowing for endless creativity in dessert preparation.

Popular Fruit-Based Delights:
Fruit Salad: A medley of fresh, ripe fruits, such as strawberries, watermelon, kiwi, and citrus, creates a colorful and refreshing dessert.

Fruit Skewers: Thread chunks of assorted fruits onto skewers for a fun and portable treat, perfect for gatherings.

Fruit Parfait: Layer Greek yogurt, granola, and fresh berries for a creamy and crunchy parfait that's as visually appealing as it is delicious.

Fruit Popsicles: Blend fruits with water or fruit juice, pour the mixture into popsicle molds, and freeze for a cooling and kid-friendly dessert.

Fruit Salsa with Cinnamon Chips: Dice fruits like apples, strawberries, and mangoes and toss them with a splash of citrus juice for a fruity salsa, served with cinnamon-sugar-dusted tortilla chips.

Berry Crumble: Combine mixed berries with a crumbly topping made from oats, flour, and a touch of sweetener for a warm and comforting dessert.

Grilled Pineapple: Grilling pineapple slices caramelizes their natural sugars, enhancing their sweetness and creating a deliciously smoky flavor.

Fruit Sorbet: Blend frozen fruits with a splash of fruit juice or yogurt to create a dairy-free and refreshing sorbet.

Fruit Tarts: Arrange slices of your favorite fruits on a pastry crust filled with custard or cream for an elegant dessert.

Baked Apples: Core and stuff apples with a mixture of oats, nuts, cinnamon, and honey before baking them until tender.

Fruit Smoothie Bowls: Blend fruits with yogurt or milk to create a creamy base, then top with granola, nuts, seeds, and more fruit for added texture and flavor.

Fruit Sushi: Roll sticky rice with fruit slices and a drizzle of honey for a playful and visually stunning dessert.

Customization and Tips:

Experiment with fruit combinations to create your own signature fruit-based delights.

Adjust the sweetness to your preference by using natural sweeteners like honey, maple syrup, or agave nectar sparingly.

Consider adding herbs like mint or basil to enhance the flavor and aroma of your fruit-based desserts.

Don't hesitate to get creative with presentation; attractive plating can elevate the enjoyment of these delightful treats.

Fruit-based delights are a celebration of nature's bounty, offering a perfect balance of sweetness, freshness, and nutrition. Whether you're making a simple fruit salad or an elaborate fruit tart, these desserts have the power to satisfy your sweet cravings while providing a wholesome and health-conscious indulgence. So, embrace the joy of fruit-based delights and savor the natural goodness that only fresh fruits can bring to your desserts.

Baked Apples with Cinnamon

Baked apples with cinnamon are a classic dessert that combines the natural sweetness of apples with the warm and aromatic flavors of cinnamon and spices. This simple yet satisfying dessert captures the essence of fall and provides a comforting and wholesome treat that's perfect for any time of year. Let's delve into why baked apples with cinnamon are so beloved and how to make this delightful dessert.

Key Ingredients:

Apples: Choose firm, sweet apples like Honeycrisp, Fuji, or Gala for the best results. The natural sweetness of these apples intensifies when baked.

Cinnamon: Ground cinnamon is the star spice that infuses the apples with warmth and flavor.

Sweetener: Options include brown sugar, maple syrup, honey, or agave nectar to add sweetness and enhance the caramelization of the apples.

Butter: A small amount of butter or a dairy-free alternative is used to add richness and prevent the apples from drying out during baking.

Why We Love Baked Apples with Cinnamon:

Comforting Aroma: The scent of baked apples and cinnamon wafting through your kitchen is like a warm hug on a chilly day.

Natural Sweetness: Baked apples are a naturally sweet dessert with no need for excessive added sugars.

Balanced Nutrition: Apples are rich in dietary fiber, vitamins, and antioxidants, making this dessert both delicious and nutritious.

Versatility: Baked apples can be enjoyed on their own, served with a scoop of vanilla ice cream, or used as a topping for oatmeal or yogurt.

How to Make Baked Apples with Cinnamon:

Here's a basic recipe to create your own Baked Apples with Cinnamon:

Ingredients:

4 apples (Honeycrisp, Fuji, or Gala work well)

2 tablespoons brown sugar (or your preferred sweetener)

1 teaspoon ground cinnamon

2 tablespoons unsalted butter (or dairy-free alternative)

Optional toppings: raisins, chopped nuts, or a honey drizzle

Instructions:

Preheat the Oven:

Preheat your oven to 375°F (190°C).

Prepare the Apples:

Wash and core the apples, removing the seeds and creating a hollow center in each apple. A paring knife or an apple corer can be used.

Mix the Filling:

In a small bowl, combine the brown sugar and ground cinnamon to create the filling mixture.

Fill the Apples:

Spoon the filling mixture evenly into the hollowed centers of the apples.

Add Butter:

Place a small pat of butter on top of the filling in each apple. This will help create a rich and buttery sauce as the apples bake.

Bake:

Arrange the filled apples in a baking dish, and bake them in the preheated oven for approximately 30-40 minutes or until the apples are tender and can be easily pierced with a fork.

Serve Warm:

Remove the baked apples from the oven, let them cool slightly, and serve them warm. Optionally, top with chopped nuts, raisins, or a drizzle of honey for added texture and flavor.

Customization:

Experiment with different sweeteners, such as maple syrup or agave nectar, to customize the level of sweetness.

Add a pinch of nutmeg or cloves to the cinnamon mixture for a more complex spice profile.

Enhance the texture with chopped nuts like walnuts or pecans, or add dried fruits like cranberries or raisins.

Baked apples with cinnamon are a comforting and wholesome dessert that encapsulates the essence of homey, fall-inspired flavors. The combination of tender, sweet apples with warm cinnamon and a touch of sweetness creates a dessert that's not only delicious but also evokes a sense of coziness and nostalgia.

Whether you're enjoying it as a family dessert or a personal indulgence, baked apples with cinnamon are sure to warm your heart and palate alike. So, embrace the simplicity and comfort of this delightful dessert, and savor each spoonful of warm, spiced goodness.

Mixed Berry Parfait

Ingredients:

1 cup of mixed berries, including blackberries, raspberries, blueberries, and strawberries

1 cup Greek yogurt or regular yogurt

1/2 cup granola

Optional sweetener (honey, maple syrup, or agave nectar)

Fresh mint leaves or extra berries for garnish (optional)

Instructions:

Prepare the Berries:

Wash and dry the berries. If using strawberries, cut them into bite-sized pieces after removing the stems.

Sweeten the Yogurt (Optional):

If your yogurt isn't already sweetened or you prefer extra sweetness, add a drizzle of honey, maple syrup, or agave nectar to the yogurt. Stir to combine.

Layer the Parfait:

Start by adding a spoonful of yogurt to the bottom of a clear glass or parfait dish.

Spread some mixed berries over the yoghurt.

Top the berries with a coating of granola.

Repeat the layers until you've used up all your ingredients, finishing with a layer of berries on top.

Garnish (Optional):

If desired, garnish your parfait with a few extra berries or fresh mint leaves for a pop of color and freshness.

Serve Immediately:

Serve your mixed berry parfait immediately to enjoy the contrasting textures and flavors at their best.

Customization:

Get creative with your parfait by adding other toppings like chopped nuts, coconut flakes, or a drizzle of fruit sauce.

Experiment with different types of yogurt, including dairy-free alternatives like almond or coconut yogurt, to suit dietary preferences.

For added sweetness and texture, consider layering with fruit preserves or compote.

Mixed berry parfaits are a celebration of nature's bounty and a testament to the joy of combining fresh, seasonal fruits with creamy yogurt and crunchy granola. Whether you're serving them for breakfast, dessert, or a special treat, these parfaits offer a burst of color, flavor, and nutrition in every bite. So, embrace the beauty and taste of mixed berry parfaits, and savor the sweet and tangy goodness that comes with each spoonful

Treats in Moderation

Treats in Moderation: Balancing Indulgence and Well-Being
"Treats in moderation" is a mantra that resonates with many, emphasizing the importance of balance in our approach to indulging in delicious, often less healthy, foods. It's a philosophy that encourages us to enjoy the pleasures of culinary delights while still maintaining a focus on overall well-being. Let's explore the significance of treats in moderation and how it can contribute to a more balanced and fulfilling lifestyle.

Understanding Treats in Moderation:

Balancing Act: Treats in moderation are about finding equilibrium between enjoying your favorite indulgent foods and making choices that prioritize your health.

Mindful Consumption: It involves being mindful of portion sizes and the frequency of consumption of treats to prevent overindulgence.

Preventing Deprivation: You can lessen the sensation of deprivation that might result in binge eating or the guilt that comes with enjoying food by permitting treats on occasion.

Savoring the Moment: It encourages you to savor each treat, enjoying it fully rather than consuming it mindlessly.

The Benefits of Treats in Moderation:

Emotional Well-Being: Treating yourself occasionally can boost your mood and provide comfort, which is essential for emotional well-being.

Sustainability: A balanced approach to treats is more sustainable over the long term, making it easier to maintain a healthy lifestyle.

Flexibility: It allows for flexibility in your diet, so you don't feel restricted or limited in your food choices.

Social Enjoyment: Treating yourself can enhance social experiences, as many gatherings and celebrations revolve around shared indulgent foods.

Practical Tips for Practicing Treats in Moderation:

Plan Ahead: Choose specific occasions or days for treats, rather than indulging impulsively.

Portion Control: Pay attention to serving sizes to prevent overindulging. Share desserts or take leftovers home when dining out.

Quality Over Quantity: Opt for high-quality treats that truly satisfy your cravings, rather than consuming empty calories from less satisfying options.

Listen to Your Body: Recognize your signs of hunger and fullness to prevent overindulging in sweets.

Stay Active: Incorporate regular physical activity into your routine to help offset the occasional indulgence.

Mindful Eating: Practice mindful eating by savoring the flavors, textures, and aromas of your treats.

Keep a Balance: Ensure that the majority of your diet consists of nutritious foods like fruits, vegetables, lean proteins, and whole grains.

Examples of Treats in Moderation:
Dark Chocolate: Enjoying a square or two of dark chocolate after dinner rather than an entire chocolate bar.

Dessert on Special Occasions: Having dessert when celebrating birthdays, holidays, or other special events.

Weekend Treats: Designating the weekends for enjoying treats like pastries, ice cream, or a favorite homemade dish.

Restaurant Dinners: Ordering a dessert when dining out but sharing it with your dining companions.

Baking at Home: Baking your favorite treats at home and enjoying them in moderation.

Snack Time: Treating yourself to a small serving of potato chips or popcorn during movie night.

Fancy Coffee: Indulging in a specialty coffee or tea drink on occasion rather than daily.

Treats in moderation are a realistic and sustainable way to strike a balance between enjoying the pleasures of food and maintaining a healthy lifestyle. It's a reminder that indulgence can coexist with well-being when approached mindfully and in a controlled manner.

Banana and Almond Butter Cookies

Banana and almond butter cookies are a delightful treat that combines the natural sweetness of ripe bananas with the rich and nutty flavors of almond butter. These cookies offer a healthier twist on traditional cookies by incorporating wholesome ingredients while still satisfying your sweet tooth. Let's explore why banana and almond butter cookies are so beloved and how to make them for your next baking adventure.

Key Ingredients:

Ripe Bananas: Overripe bananas are the star of the show, providing natural sweetness and moisture to the cookies.

Almond Butter: Almond butter adds nuttiness, creaminess, and a dose of healthy fats to the cookies.

Oats: Rolled oats provide texture, fiber, and heartiness to the cookies.

Sweetener: A touch of honey, maple syrup, or a natural sweetener of your choice is used to enhance the sweetness of the cookies.

Spices: The flavors of vanilla essence, nutmeg, and cinnamon give warmth and complexity.

Why We Love Banana and Almond Butter Cookies:
Healthier Alternative: These cookies offer a nutritious twist on traditional cookies by using whole ingredients and natural sweeteners.

Quick and Easy: The recipe is simple and requires minimal time and effort, making it perfect for both novice and experienced bakers.

Gluten-Free Option: If you use gluten-free oats, these cookies can be suitable for a gluten-free diet.

Kid-Friendly: Kids love the natural sweetness of bananas, making these cookies a hit with little ones.

How to Make Banana and Almond Butter Cookies:

Here's a basic recipe to create your own Banana and Almond Butter Cookies:

Ingredients:

2 ripe bananas, mashed

1/2 cup almond butter

1 1/2 cups rolled oats

2 tablespoons honey or maple syrup

1/2 teaspoon cinnamon

1/4 teaspoon nutmeg

1/2 teaspoon vanilla extract

A pinch of salt

Instructions:

Preheat the Oven:

Preheat your oven to 350°F (175°C). Use parchment paper to line a baking sheet.

Mix Wet Ingredients:

In a mixing bowl, combine the mashed bananas, almond butter, honey or maple syrup, and vanilla extract. Mix until smooth.

Add Dry Ingredients:

Add the rolled oats, cinnamon, nutmeg, and a pinch of salt to the wet ingredients. Mixing the components thoroughly requires stirring.

Scoop and Shape:

Using a spoon or cookie scoop, drop spoonsful of the cookie dough onto the prepared baking sheet, spacing them a couple of inches apart.

Flatten Slightly:

Gently flatten each cookie with the back of a fork or the palm of your hand.

Bake:

Bake in the preheated oven for 10-12 minutes, or until the cookies are set and the edges turn golden brown.

Cool and Enjoy:

After a few minutes of cooling on the baking sheet, move the cookies to a wire rack to finish cooling.

Store: Store any leftover cookies in an airtight container at room temperature for up to a few days.

Customization:

Get creative by adding your favorite mix-ins like chocolate chips, chopped nuts, or dried fruits to the cookie dough.

Experiment with different nut or seed butters like peanut butter, cashew butter, or sunflower seed butter.

Adjust the sweetness by using more or less honey or maple syrup to suit your taste.

Banana and almond butter cookies are a wholesome and delicious treat that brings together the comforting flavors of ripe bananas and nutty almond butter. They are perfect for a quick snack, a healthy dessert, or a grab-and-go breakfast option. By incorporating simple, natural ingredients, these cookies allow you to indulge in a sweet treat while still making mindful choices for your well-being. So, embrace the nutty sweetness of these cookies and enjoy a guilt-free delight with each bite.

Rice Pudding with a Twist

Rice pudding is a beloved dessert known for its comforting, creamy texture and gentle sweetness. While the classic recipe is cherished by many, sometimes it's fun to give traditional dishes a creative twist. In this exploration of rice pudding with a twist, we'll dive into how to take this timeless treat to new heights of flavor and delight.

The Classic Rice Pudding:

Before we delve into the twists, let's briefly explore the basics of classic rice pudding:

Ingredients:

Arborio rice or medium-grain rice

Milk (whole milk, evaporated milk, or coconut milk)

Sugar

Vanilla extract

Cinnamon

Raisins (optional)

A pinch of salt

Cooking Process:

Rinse the rice and cook it in milk until the rice is tender and the mixture thickens.

Sweeten with sugar and add a dash of vanilla extract for flavor.

Enhance with cinnamon and, if desired, raisins for added sweetness and texture.

Serve warm or cold, topped with a dollop of whipped cream or a sprinkling of cinnamon.

Rice Pudding Twists:

Now, let's explore some creative twists you can apply to your rice pudding:

Chocolate Lover's Delight: Stir in cocoa powder or melted dark chocolate for a rich and indulgent chocolate rice pudding. Add some chocolate sauce or chocolate shavings on top.

Fruit Fusion: Incorporate diced fresh fruits like mango, pineapple, or berries for a burst of freshness and a tropical twist to your rice pudding.

Citrus Zest: Add grated orange or lemon zest to infuse your rice pudding with citrusy brightness. A splash of citrus juice can also provide a tangy contrast.

Nutty Crunch: Sprinkle chopped nuts like almonds, pistachios, or pecans on top for added texture and a delightful nutty flavor.

Spice It Up: Experiment with spices like cardamom, nutmeg, or chai spice blends for a more complex and aromatic flavor profile.

Coconut Dream: Swap some or all of the milk with coconut milk to create a creamy and tropical coconut rice pudding. Top with toasted coconut flakes for extra crunch.

Savory Surprise: Transform your rice pudding into a savory side dish by reducing the sugar and incorporating ingredients like

Parmesan cheese, saffron, and sautéed onions for a unique twist on a classic comfort food.

Caramelized Banana Bliss: Sauté sliced bananas in brown sugar and butter until caramelized, then fold them into your rice pudding for a sweet and gooey surprise.

Matcha Magic: Infuse your rice pudding with matcha green tea powder for a vibrant green color and earthy, slightly bitter notes. Add some whipped cream and matcha powder over top.

Tropical Escape: Mix in shredded coconut, diced pineapple, and a splash of rum extract to create a tropical rice pudding reminiscent of a piña colada.

Presentation and Garnish:
Don't forget the importance of presentation. A sprinkle of ground cinnamon, a drizzle of honey, or a dollop of whipped cream can transform your rice pudding into an elegant dessert. Serve it in individual ramekins, glass jars, or small dessert bowls to make it visually appealing.

Rice pudding with a twist allows you to infuse your own personality and creativity into a classic dessert. By experimenting with different ingredients, flavors, and textures, you can take this comforting treat to new heights and surprise your taste buds with exciting variations. Whether you're a fan of chocolate, fruit, spices, or nuts, there's a rice pudding twist waiting for you to discover and enjoy.

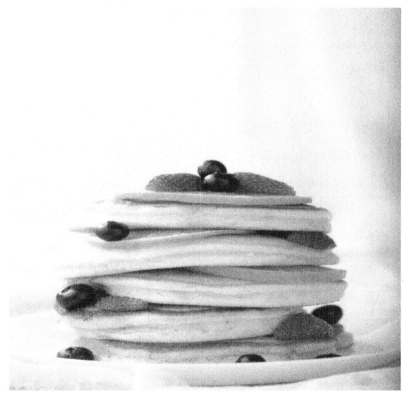

Chapter 6

Special Occasions and Dining Out

Special occasions provide the perfect opportunity to indulge in culinary delights and create memorable dining experiences. Whether you're celebrating a birthday, anniversary, holiday, or simply treating yourself to a night out, making thoughtful choices about where and what to eat can elevate the occasion. Let's explore how to make the most of special occasions when dining out.

Choosing the Right Restaurant:

Consider the Atmosphere: Select a restaurant that aligns with the ambiance you desire for the occasion. Whether it's a cozy and intimate setting or a lively and vibrant atmosphere, the right environment can enhance the experience.

Cuisine Preferences: Take into account the preferences of everyone dining with you. Opt for a restaurant that offers a variety of dishes to cater to different tastes and dietary restrictions.

Reservations: Special occasions often mean busy restaurants. Make a reservation well in advance to secure your preferred dining time and avoid disappointment.

Read Reviews: Research online reviews and ask for recommendations from friends or family to ensure the restaurant meets your expectations in terms of food quality and service.

Choosing Your Meal:
Explore the Menu: Special occasions are an opportunity to explore and try something new. Consider ordering dishes you haven't tried before or selecting the chef's tasting menu for a curated culinary journey.

Indulge Wisely: While indulgence is part of the special occasion experience, balance it with mindful choices. If you plan to have a rich dessert, consider ordering a lighter main course.

Share Plates: Sharing appetizers, entrees, and desserts can allow you to taste a variety of dishes and make the meal feel even more special.

Dining Etiquette:

Dress Accordingly: Dressing up for the occasion adds to the sense of importance and makes the meal feel more special.

Be Punctual: Arriving on time shows respect for the restaurant staff and allows you to make the most of your reservation.

Mindful Dining: Put away distractions like phones and focus on the meal and the company you're with. Talk to each other and enjoy every bite.

Wine and Beverage Choices:

Wine Pairing: If you're having wine with your meal, consider asking for wine pairings or consulting the sommelier for recommendations that complement your food choices.

Non-Alcoholic Options: For those who prefer non-alcoholic beverages, many restaurants offer creative and sophisticated mocktails.

Dessert and Celebration:

Celebrate with Dessert: Conclude your meal with a special dessert to mark the occasion. Consider sharing a dessert sampler to taste a variety of sweet treats.

Bring Your Own Cake: Some restaurants allow you to bring your own cake or dessert for special occasions. Inquire in advance if this is an option.

Express Gratitude:

Thank the Staff: Show appreciation to the restaurant staff for their service. A kind word or a gratuity that reflects the exceptional service can go a long way.

Safety and Health Considerations:

Allergies and Dietary Restrictions: If anyone in your party has food allergies or dietary restrictions, communicate these clearly to the restaurant staff when making reservations and ordering.

COVID-19 Protocols: Stay informed about the restaurant's COVID-19 safety measures and comply with any requirements, such as mask-wearing or vaccine mandates.

Dining out on special occasions is an opportunity to create cherished memories and indulge in exceptional cuisine. By selecting the right restaurant, making thoughtful choices about your meal, and practicing dining etiquette, you can make the experience even more memorable. Whether you're celebrating with loved ones or treating yourself, savoring the moment and enjoying the culinary journey can make special occasions truly unforgettable.

Celebratory Meals

Celebratory meals hold a unique place in our lives. They mark important milestones, strengthen bonds with loved ones, and allow us to savor life's special moments. Whether you're celebrating a birthday, anniversary, graduation, promotion, or any other significant event, the act of coming together around a delicious meal enhances the joy of the occasion. Let's explore the art of celebratory meals and how to make them truly memorable.

The Essence of Celebratory Meals:

Gathering and Connection: Celebratory meals are a way to bring people together. They create a sense of togetherness and allow friends and family to connect and share in the joy of the moment.

Creating Memories: These meals are often remembered not only for the food but also for the shared laughter, heartfelt conversations, and the warmth of being surrounded by loved ones.

Reflecting on Achievements: Celebratory meals are an opportunity to reflect on and celebrate achievements, milestones, and the journey that led to this special moment.

Tips for Planning Celebratory Meals:

Selecting the Venue: Choose a venue that aligns with the tone and significance of the celebration. This could be a fine-dining restaurant, a cozy family-owned bistro, a scenic picnic spot, or even your own home.

Personalize the Menu: Consider personalizing the menu to reflect the preferences of the guest of honor. Incorporate their favorite dishes or cuisines, or explore new culinary experiences together.

Toast to Success: Raise a toast to celebrate the occasion. Whether it's with champagne, wine, sparkling cider, or a special cocktail, toasting adds a sense of ceremony.

Decorate Thoughtfully: Enhance the atmosphere with decorations that reflect the theme or purpose of the celebration. Flowers, candles, and personalized place settings can make the meal feel more special.

Plan Surprise Elements: Consider adding surprise elements to the meal, such as a heartfelt speech, a slideshow of memorable moments, or a small gift that holds sentimental value.

Menu Ideas for Celebratory Meals:

Multi-Course Feast: A multi-course meal with appetizers, soup or salad, a main course, and dessert is a classic choice for formal celebrations.

Tasting Menu: Explore a tasting menu at a renowned restaurant for a culinary adventure that showcases a variety of flavors and techniques.

Cultural Experience: Celebrate with cuisine from a specific culture or region, immersing yourself in the flavors and traditions of that place.

Outdoor Picnic: For a casual celebration, opt for an outdoor picnic with an array of finger foods, sandwiches, and refreshing beverages.

Cooking Together: Gather family and friends for a cooking session where everyone participates in preparing the celebratory meal.

Potluck Gathering: Encourage guests to bring dishes they love for a potluck-style celebration, creating a diverse and delicious spread.

The Gift of Presence:

While the food and ambiance are important, it's the presence of loved ones that truly makes celebratory meals special. Engage in meaningful conversations, share stories, and take the time to express gratitude and love for one another.

Capture the Moment:

Consider documenting the occasion with photos or a journal. These keepsakes will allow you to relive the joy of the celebration in the years to come.

Express Gratitude:

Take a moment during the celebratory meal to express gratitude for the people who have been a part of the journey leading up to this special moment. We appreciate their attendance and assistance.

Celebratory meals are a cherished tradition that adds depth and meaning to life's milestones. They offer an opportunity to pause, appreciate our achievements, and connect with those who matter most. By planning thoughtfully and savoring the experience, you can make these meals a beautiful and lasting memory that you and your loved ones will treasure for years to come.

Grilled Shrimp and Vegetable Skewers

Grilled shrimp and vegetable skewers are the epitome of summer dining—a feast of vibrant colors, fresh flavors, and the irresistible aroma of food sizzling on the grill. These skewers offer a delightful combination of succulent shrimp and a rainbow of seasonal vegetables, all seasoned to perfection. Let's dive into the world of grilled shrimp and vegetable skewers and discover why they are a favorite during the warm months.

Key Ingredients:

Shrimp: Use large, peeled, and deveined shrimp for convenience. They cook quickly and absorb the flavors of your marinade beautifully.

Vegetables: Opt for a variety of colorful vegetables such as bell peppers, red onions, cherry tomatoes, zucchini, and mushrooms. This diversity adds visual appeal and a range of flavors and textures.

Marinade: Create a simple yet flavorful marinade with ingredients like olive oil, garlic, lemon juice, herbs (like parsley or cilantro), and your choice of spices or seasonings (e.g., paprika, cayenne, or Italian seasoning).

Skewers: Wooden or metal skewers work, but if using wooden ones, soak them in water for at least 30 minutes before threading the ingredients to prevent burning on the grill.

Why We Love Grilled Shrimp and Vegetable Skewers:
Balanced and Nutritious: These skewers offer a balanced meal with lean protein from shrimp and an array of vitamins, minerals, and fiber from the vegetables.

Customizable: You can personalize the skewers by using your favorite vegetables and adjusting the seasonings to your taste.

Quick and Easy: Grilling ensures that the skewers cook quickly, making them a perfect choice for weeknight dinners or outdoor gatherings.

Versatile Presentation: Grilled skewers are visually appealing and can be served as a main course or appetizer.

How to Prepare Vegetable and Shrimp Skewers on the Grill:
Here's a basic recipe to create your own Grilled Shrimp and Vegetable Skewers:

Ingredients:
1-pound large shrimp, peeled and deveined
2 colorful bell peppers, chopped into bits
1 red onion, cut into chunks
1 zucchini, sliced into rounds
Cherry tomatoes
8-10 cremini mushrooms, cleaned and stems removed
Wooden or metal skewers
3 tablespoons olive oil
2 cloves garlic, minced

Juice of 1 lemon

1 tablespoon fresh parsley, chopped

Salt and pepper to taste

Optional: Your choice of seasoning (e.g., paprika, cayenne, or Italian seasoning)

Instructions:

Prepare the Marinade:

In a bowl, whisk together olive oil, minced garlic, lemon juice, chopped parsley, and your choice of seasoning. Add salt and pepper to taste.

Marinate the Shrimp:

Transfer the prawns to another bowl and cover them with half of the marinade. Toss to coat evenly and let them marinate for about 15-20 minutes in the refrigerator.

Thread the Skewers:

Preheat your grill to medium-high heat.

Thread the marinated shrimp, bell peppers, red onions, zucchini, cherry tomatoes, and mushrooms onto the skewers in alternating order.

Grill the Skewers:

Brush the skewers with the remaining marinade.

Grill the skewers for 2-3 minutes per side or until the shrimp turn pink and the vegetables are charred and tender.

Serve Hot:

Serve the skewers hot after transferring them to a serving plate.

Optionally, garnish with extra chopped parsley and lemon wedges.

Customization:

Feel free to add your favorite vegetables or switch out the shrimp for other proteins like chicken, tofu, or even beef if you prefer.

Experiment with different marinade ingredients to create a unique flavor profile, such as adding soy sauce, honey, or Dijon mustard.

Grilled shrimp and vegetable skewers are a celebration of summer's bounty and the joys of outdoor grilling. Whether you're enjoying them on a weeknight or as part of a weekend barbecue, these skewers are sure to be a hit with their combination of tender shrimp and charred, flavorful vegetables. So, fire up the grill, savor the smoky aroma, and relish every bite of this delightful summertime dish.

Quinoa-Stuffed Bell Peppers

Quinoa-stuffed bell peppers are a delightful and nutritious meal that combines the nutty goodness of quinoa with the vibrant flavors of bell peppers and a medley of vegetables. This vegetarian dish is not only visually appealing but also packed with essential nutrients and protein. Whether you're a vegetarian or simply looking for a delicious and wholesome meal, quinoa-stuffed bell peppers are a fantastic option. Let's explore why these stuffed peppers are so popular and how to make them yourself.

Key Ingredients:

Bell Peppers: Choose firm, large bell peppers in various colors to add a visually appealing and diverse flavor profile.

Quinoa: Quinoa is the star of the stuffing, offering a complete source of protein, fiber, and essential vitamins and minerals.

Vegetables: The stuffing can include a variety of vegetables such as onions, garlic, tomatoes, corn, peas, and spinach for added texture, flavor, and nutrition.

Seasonings and Herbs: Utilize a blend of seasonings like cumin, paprika, and chili powder for depth of flavor. Fresh herbs like parsley or cilantro can also enhance the dish.

Cheese (optional): If you're not strictly vegan, a sprinkle of cheese on top adds a creamy and savory element to the dish.

Why We Love Quinoa-Stuffed Bell Peppers:

Balanced Nutrition: Quinoa offers a high-quality protein source and is packed with fiber, making these stuffed peppers a balanced and satisfying meal.

Vibrant Presentation: The colorful bell peppers, when stuffed and baked, create an attractive and inviting dish that's perfect for special occasions or everyday dining.

Customizable: You can customize the stuffing with your favorite vegetables and seasonings, making it a versatile option for various tastes and dietary preferences.

Healthy and Wholesome: This dish is a nutritious choice that fits into vegetarian, vegan, gluten-free, and dairy-free diets.

How to Make Quinoa-Stuffed Bell Peppers:

Here's a basic recipe to create your own Quinoa-Stuffed Bell Peppers:

Ingredients:

4 large bell peppers (red, green, yellow, or orange)

1 cup quinoa, rinsed and drained

2 cups vegetable broth or water

1 tablespoon olive oil

1 small onion, finely chopped

2 cloves garlic, minced

1 cup diced tomatoes (fresh or canned)

1 cup mixed vegetables (e.g., corn, peas, diced carrots)

1 teaspoon ground cumin

1 teaspoon paprika

1/2 teaspoon chili powder (adjust to taste)

Salt and pepper to taste

Fresh herbs (e.g., parsley or cilantro) for garnish

Grated cheese (optional)

Instructions:

Prepare the Bell Peppers:

Slice off the bell peppers' tops, then take out the seeds and membranes. Put the tops away for later. Sprinkle a small amount of salt and pepper inside the peppers.

Cook the Quinoa:

In a saucepan, combine the quinoa and vegetable broth (or water) and bring to a boil. Once the quinoa is cooked and the liquid has been absorbed, lower the heat, cover, and simmer for 15 to 20 minutes.

Prepare the Stuffing:

Heat the olive oil in a pan over medium heat. Add the minced garlic and onion, and cook until transparent and aromatic.

Stir in the diced tomatoes, mixed vegetables, ground cumin, paprika, chili powder, salt, and pepper. Simmer the veggies for a few minutes, or until they are soft.

Add the cooked quinoa to the skillet and stir to combine all the ingredients. Adjust the seasoning if needed.

Stuff the Peppers:

Preheat your oven to 375°F (190°C).

Stuff each bell pepper with the quinoa and vegetable mixture, pressing down gently to ensure they are well-packed.

Bake:

The stuffed bell peppers should be put on a baking dish. Garnish each pepper with grated cheese, if you'd like.

Bake the peppers in the baking dish for 25 to 30 minutes, or until they are soft, covered with aluminum foil.

Garnish and Serve:

Remove the foil and bake for an additional 5-10 minutes until the cheese (if used) is melted and golden.

Garnish the stuffed peppers with fresh herbs like parsley or cilantro before serving.

Customization:

You can add protein to the stuffing by incorporating cooked lentils, black beans, or chickpeas.

Try varying the spices and seasonings to produce different flavor profiles.

For a spicy kick, consider adding diced jalapeños or red pepper flakes.

Quinoa-stuffed bell peppers are a wholesome and satisfying meal that celebrates the harmony of fresh vegetables, quinoa's nutritional powerhouse, and a burst of seasonings. Whether served as a main course or side dish, this dish is a crowd-pleaser that brings together health-conscious eating and delightful flavors. So, gather your ingredients, stuff those colorful peppers, and enjoy a flavorful, wholesome feast that celebrates the beauty of nature's bounty.

Navigating Restaurant Menus

Dining out at a restaurant can be a delightful experience, offering a break from cooking and a chance to enjoy a variety of cuisines.

However, restaurant menus often tempt us with a wide array of dishes, making it challenging to make healthy and balanced choices. Learning how to navigate restaurant menus effectively can help you enjoy your meal while still making mindful choices for your health and well-being. The following advice will help you get the most out of your eating experience:

1. **Review the Menu in Advance:**
Many restaurants post their menus online, allowing you to review them before your visit. Take advantage of this opportunity to plan your meal in advance. Find meals that fit your dietary preferences and health objectives.

2. Scan the Menu Strategically:

When you're at the restaurant, take a moment to scan the menu strategically:

Appetizers: Consider starting with a salad, broth-based soup, or a vegetable-based appetizer. These options can help curb your appetite and provide essential nutrients.

Main Course: Look for dishes that incorporate lean protein sources like chicken, fish, tofu, or legumes. Opt for grilled, baked, or steamed preparations over fried or breaded options.

Side Dishes: Choose sides that feature vegetables, whole grains, or salads instead of heavy starches or fried options.

Beverages: Drink water or opt for unsweetened beverages like herbal tea, sparkling water, or a small glass of wine if you prefer alcohol. Avoid sugary sodas and excessive cocktails.

3. Be Mindful of Portion Sizes:

Restaurant portions are often larger than what you might eat at home. Consider sharing an entrée with a dining companion or ask for a to-go container to pack up half your meal before you start eating. This can help prevent overeating and allow you to enjoy the leftovers later.

4. Customize Your Order:

Please feel free to alter your order to accommodate any dietary restrictions. Ask for dressings or sauces on the side, request steamed or sautéed vegetables instead of fries, and choose whole grain options when available.

5. Be Wary of Hidden Ingredients:

Some restaurant dishes may contain hidden sources of added sugars, unhealthy fats, or excessive sodium. Ask your server about ingredient details or preparation methods if you have specific dietary concerns.

6. **Watch Out for "Health Halos":**

Beware of dishes that are labeled as "healthy" or "light." These labels can sometimes be misleading. Review the ingredients and nutritional information to ensure they align with your dietary goals.

7. **Balance Your Meal:**

Aim for a balanced meal that includes a source of lean protein, plenty of vegetables, and a small serving of whole grains or other complex carbohydrates. This balance helps provide essential nutrients and keeps you feeling satisfied.

8. **Practice Portion Control:**

Consider splitting a dessert with your dining companions if you'd like to indulge in something sweet. Alternatively, choose a dessert option that is smaller or lower in calories, such as a fruit-based dessert or a sorbet.

9. Listen to Your Body:

Observe the signals your body sends when it is hungry or full. Eat slowly and savor each bite. Instead of eating everything on your plate, stop eating when you're satisfied.

10. Enjoy the Experience:

Eating out is about more than simply the cuisine; it's about the whole experience. Enjoy the ambiance, the company of friends or family, and the opportunity to try new flavors and cuisines in a social setting.

Navigating restaurant menus can be a rewarding experience when you make informed choices that align with your health and taste preferences. By scanning the menu strategically, customizing your order, and practicing portion control, you can enjoy dining out while also prioritizing your well-being. Remember that moderation and mindfulness are key to finding balance between indulgence and healthy choices when dining at restaurants.

Tips for Ordering at Restaurants

Ordering at restaurants can be a pleasurable experience, offering an opportunity to savor a variety of cuisines and flavors. However, it can also be a challenge when trying to make healthy and mindful choices. Whether you're dining out for a special occasion or grabbing a quick meal, these tips can help you navigate restaurant menus and make choices that align with your dietary preferences and wellness goals.

1. Plan Ahead:

Check the Menu Online: Many restaurants now post their menus online. Take a look in advance to familiarize yourself with the options and consider what suits your dietary needs.

2. Consider the Cuisine:

Explore Ethnic Cuisines: Ethnic restaurants often offer a variety of dishes with fresh ingredients, herbs, and spices. Mediterranean, Japanese, Thai, and Greek cuisines often feature healthier options.

3. Start with Soup or Salad:

Appetizers: Begin your meal with a soup, salad, or a vegetable-based appetizer. This can help fill you up with nutrient-rich foods and curb your appetite for the main course.

4. Choose Lean Proteins:

Protein Selection: Opt for lean protein sources like grilled chicken, turkey, fish, tofu, legumes, or lean cuts of beef. Avoid fried or heavily breaded options.

5. Beware of Hidden Calories:

Sauces and Dressings: Be cautious of calorie-laden sauces and dressings. To help you manage how much you use, ask to have them on the side.

6. Customize Your Order:

Special Requests: Don't hesitate to make special requests, such as substituting fries for a side salad or asking for a smaller portion.

7. Mind the Sides:

Choose Wisely: Opt for healthier side dishes like steamed or roasted vegetables, quinoa, brown rice, or a sweet potato instead of fries or mashed potatoes.

8. Be Wary of Portions:

Portion Control: Restaurant servings are frequently greater than required. Consider sharing an entrée or asking for a to-go box to save leftovers.

9. Hydrate Smartly:

Drink Water: Begin your meal with a glass of water, and continue to hydrate throughout your meal. By doing this, you may manage your hunger and avoid overindulging.

10. Watch Alcohol Consumption:

Moderate Alcohol: If you choose to consume alcohol, do so in moderation. Stick to one drink and avoid excessive cocktails with sugary mixers.

11. Listen to Your Body:

Hunger Cues: Recognize the signs of hunger and fullness sent by your body. Eat mindfully, slowly, and stop when you're satisfied but not full. Savor every bite.

12. Share Desserts:

Indulge Smartly: If you want dessert, consider sharing it with your dining companions to enjoy a sweet treat without overindulging.

13. Be Mindful:

Stay Mindful: Stay present during your meal. Put away distractions like phones and engage in conversation with your dining companions.

14. Don't Be Too Hard on Yourself:

Occasional Indulgence: Remember that it's okay to enjoy indulgent meals occasionally. Dining out is also about the experience and enjoying flavors.

15. Practice Flexibility:

Flexibility is Key: While it's important to make healthy choices, be flexible when dining out. It's okay to enjoy your favorite dish on occasion, but balance it with healthier choices in other meals.

Navigating restaurant menus can be a rewarding experience when you prioritize both taste and nutrition. By planning ahead, choosing wisely, and being mindful of your choices, you can enjoy dining out while staying on track with your dietary goals. Remember that balance and moderation are key to savoring the pleasures of restaurant dining while maintaining a healthy lifestyle.

Stomach-Friendly Restaurant Options

If you're dealing with stomach sensitivities or digestive issues, dining out at restaurants can be a bit tricky. However, with some knowledge and strategy, you can still enjoy restaurant meals without discomfort.

Here's a guide to finding and ordering stomach-friendly options at restaurants:

1. Choose the Right Restaurant:
Research Ahead: Look for restaurants that offer lighter, milder, or customizable dishes that are gentle on the stomach. Health-focused eateries, salad bars, sushi restaurants, and places with customizable bowls or plates can be good choices.

2. Start with a Gentle Appetizer:
Soup: A warm broth-based soup like chicken noodle, vegetable, or miso can be soothing and easy on the stomach.

Salad: Opt for a simple garden salad with fresh vegetables and a light vinaigrette dressing. Avoid salads with rich, creamy dressings or spicy ingredients.

3. Choose Lean Protein:
Protein: Lean protein sources like grilled chicken, turkey, fish, tofu, or even lean cuts of beef are often easier to digest than fatty or fried options.

4. Be Mindful of Seasonings and Sauces:

Request Sauces on the Side: Ask for any sauces or dressings to be served on the side, so you can control how much you use.

Avoid Spicy and Heavy Seasonings: Steer clear of dishes with heavy spices, garlic, onion, or chili if these tend to trigger your stomach discomfort.

5. Opt for Simple Sides:

Starchy Sides: Choose mild, starchy sides like mashed potatoes, plain rice, or a baked sweet potato. These can help settle your stomach.

Steamed Vegetables: Request steamed or lightly sautéed vegetables as a side dish. Avoid those cooked with excessive butter or oil.

6. Hydrate Wisely:

Drink Water: Start your meal with a glass of water and continue to sip throughout. Avoid carbonated or sugary beverages, as they can contribute to stomach discomfort.

7. Practice Portion Control:

Share or Save: Consider sharing an entrée or asking for a to-go box to portion your meal appropriately.

8. Choose Desserts Carefully:

Fruit-Based Desserts: Opt for fruit-based desserts or sorbet, which are often easier on the stomach than rich, heavy options.

Skip Rich and Creamy: Avoid desserts with heavy cream, chocolate, or layers of frosting if these tend to upset your stomach.

9. Communicate Dietary Restrictions:

Allergies or Intolerances: Don't hesitate to communicate your dietary restrictions or sensitivities to your server. They can help guide you to suitable menu choices or check with the kitchen regarding ingredient substitutions.

10. Practice Mindful Eating:

Slow Down: Eat slowly and mindfully. Savor each bite and pay attention to your body's signals of fullness.

11. Keep Over-the-Counter Remedies Handy:

Carry Medications: If you have prescribed or over-the-counter medications or remedies for stomach discomfort, keep them in your bag or pocket just in case.

12. Stay Relaxed:

Relaxation Techniques: Before and during your meal, practice deep breathing or other relaxation techniques to reduce stress, which can exacerbate stomach issues.

Remember that everyone's stomach sensitivity is different, so it's essential to know your triggers and be proactive in choosing foods that align with your comfort and well-being. Don't be afraid to make special requests or inquire about menu ingredients to ensure your dining experience is as enjoyable as possible. With a bit of planning and a thoughtful approach, you can continue to savor delicious restaurant meals while taking care of your stomach.

Chapter 7

Managing Stress and Lifestyle Choices

We live in a fast-paced world where stress is a common occurrence. Balancing work, family, social commitments, and personal goals can often lead to high levels of stress. However, how we manage stress and make lifestyle choices significantly impacts our overall well-being.

Here are some key strategies for effectively managing stress and making healthier lifestyle choices.

1. **Understand Stress:**

Recognize Stressors: Identify the sources of stress in your life. This might include work demands, relationship issues, financial concerns, or health challenges.

Types of Stress: Differentiate between acute stress (short-term, immediate stressors) and chronic stress (long-term, ongoing stressors).

2. **Practice Stress Management Techniques:**

Deep Breathing: Include deep breathing techniques in your everyday routine. Deep, mindful breaths can help calm your nervous system and reduce stress.

Meditation and Mindfulness: Regular meditation or mindfulness practices can increase your ability to manage stress by promoting relaxation and self-awareness.

Physical Activity: Engage in regular physical activity, which releases endorphins and helps reduce stress. Activities like yoga, tai chi, or even a simple walk can be effective.

Journaling: Keep a notebook where you can record your feelings and thoughts. This can help you process emotions and gain insight into stress triggers.

Time Management: Organize your schedule and prioritize tasks to reduce the feeling of being overwhelmed.

3. Make Healthy Diet Choices:

Eat a well-balanced diet that includes lots of fruits, vegetables, whole grains, lean meats, and healthy fats. Avoid excessive sugar, processed foods, and excessive caffeine or alcohol.

Hydration: Drink lots of water throughout the day to stay hydrated.

4. Prioritize Sleep:

Sleep Quality: Aim for seven to nine hours of good sleep every night. Establish a relaxing evening ritual and stick to a regular sleep schedule.

Limit Screen Time: Limit your time spent in front of devices (computers, tablets, and phones) before bed because the blue light they create can disrupt your sleep.

5. Foster Supportive Relationships:

Social Connections: Build and maintain meaningful relationships with friends and family. Having a support network can help you navigate stressful situations.

Open Communication: Talk to loved ones about your stressors and feelings. Sharing your concerns can provide emotional relief and lead to solutions.

6. Set Realistic Goals:

Realistic Expectations: Set achievable goals for yourself, both personally and professionally. Unnecessary tension might result from unrealistic expectations.

7. Engage in Leisure Activities:

Hobbies: Make time for activities you enjoy, whether it's reading, painting, gardening, or playing a musical instrument. Hobbies can be relaxing and give you a sense of fulfilment.

8. Seek Professional Help:

Counseling or Therapy: If you find it challenging to manage stress on your own, consider seeking the help of a mental health professional. Therapy or counseling can provide effective strategies for stress management.

Medical Evaluation: If you believe your stress is affecting your physical health, consult a healthcare provider to rule out underlying medical conditions.

9. Practice Self-Compassion:

Be Kind to Yourself: Strive for self-compassion and refrain from self-criticism. You should be kind and understanding to yourself just as you would a friend.

10. Maintain Work-Life Balance:

Set Boundaries: Define distinct boundaries between your personal and professional lives. In order to refuel during your own time, disconnect from work-related responsibilities.

11. Learn to Say No:

Manage Commitments: Don't overcommit yourself. Politely decline additional responsibilities or obligations when you need to prioritize your well-being.

12. **Stay Informed:**

Health Education: Stay informed about health and well-being by reading books, articles, or attending workshops on stress management and healthy lifestyle choices.

Managing stress and making healthier lifestyle choices is an ongoing process that requires dedication and self-awareness. By incorporating these strategies into your daily life, you can reduce stress, enhance your overall well-being, and build resilience to cope with life's challenges. Remember that it's okay to seek support when needed and that small, consistent changes can lead to significant improvements in your quality of life.

Stress-Reduction Techniques

Stress has become a regular companion in our fast-paced world of today. From work deadlines to personal responsibilities, stressors can feel overwhelming at times. However, there are effective stress-reduction techniques that can help you find calm and regain control over your well-being. Here are some proven methods to reduce stress and promote relaxation:

1. Deep Breathing:

Simple yet effective techniques for stress management are deep breathing exercises. When you practice deep breathing, you engage your body's relaxation response, which can help reduce stress hormones like cortisol.

Technique: Find a quiet space. Inhale slowly through your nose for a count of four, hold for a count of four, and exhale slowly through your mouth for a count of six. Repeat several times until you feel more relaxed.

2. Meditation:

Meditation is a practice that involves focusing your mind on a particular object, thought, or activity to train your attention and awareness. It can lessen tension and enhance mental health.

Technique: Find a comfortable, quiet place to sit or lie down. Close your eyes and focus on your breath, a mantra, or a guided meditation app. Give up on distracting ideas and focus on the here and now.

3. Mindfulness:

Being mindful entails focusing on the here and now without passing judgement. It can help you become more aware of your thoughts and feelings and reduce the impact of stressors.

Practice: Throughout your day, take a few moments to pause and observe your surroundings, thoughts, and sensations. Be fully present in whatever you're doing, whether it's eating, walking, or working.

4. Physical Activity:

Regular physical activity is a potent stress reducer. Exercise releases endorphins, which are natural mood lifters and stress relievers.

Routine: Incorporate physical activity into your daily routine, whether it's through walking, jogging, yoga, or dancing. Find something you enjoy doing and turn it into a long-lasting habit.

5. Progressive Muscle Relaxation:

Progressive muscle relaxation involves tensing and then relaxing various muscle groups in your body to release physical tension and stress.

Technique: Start with your toes and work your way up through your body, tensing each muscle group for a few seconds and then releasing. Focus on the sensations of relaxation as you do this.

6. Journaling:

Expressing your thoughts and feelings through journaling can be a therapeutic way to manage stress. It allows you to gain insight into your emotions and reduce their impact.

Process: Set aside a few minutes each day to write freely about your thoughts and emotions. No need to edit or censor; just let your thoughts flow onto the page.

7. Time Management:

Effective time management can reduce stress by helping you prioritize tasks, set realistic goals, and create a sense of control over your schedule.

Tools: Use to-do lists, calendars, and time management apps to organize your tasks and allocate time wisely.

8. Social Connections:

Spending time with friends and loved ones can provide emotional support and a sense of belonging, which can help reduce stress.

Reach Out: Make an effort to connect with friends and family regularly, whether through phone calls, video chats, or in-person gatherings.

9. Relaxation Techniques:

Engage in relaxation techniques such as taking a warm bath, practicing aromatherapy, or listening to soothing music to create a calm and serene atmosphere.

Self-Care: Set aside time for self-care activities that help you unwind and recharge.

10. **Seek Professional Help:**

If you find that stress is significantly impacting your life and well-being, don't hesitate to seek support from a mental health professional. Therapy or counseling can provide you with effective stress management strategies and tools tailored to your specific needs.

Keep in mind that stress management is a continuous process, and what suits one individual may not suit another. Experiment with different techniques to find the ones that resonate with you and fit your lifestyle. By incorporating these stress-reduction techniques into your daily routine, you can find greater peace, resilience, and well-being in the face of life's challenges.

Mindful Eating and Relaxation

In today's fast-paced world, mealtime often becomes a hurried and stressful experience. Many of us eat on the go, in front of screens, or while multitasking, which can lead to overeating, poor digestion, and a lack of appreciation for the food we consume. Mindful eating is a practice that invites us to slow down, savor each bite, and cultivate a deeper connection with our food. When combined with relaxation techniques, it can transform your relationship with food and nourish both your body and soul.

What is Mindful Eating?

A mindfulness practice called mindful eating entails giving your entire attention to the dining experience. It encourages you to be present in the moment, engage all your senses, and fully appreciate the food in front of you. By savoring each bite and listening to your body's hunger and fullness cues, mindful eating can lead to a healthier relationship with food and a greater sense of satisfaction.

How to Practice Mindful Eating:

Set the Stage: Establish a serene and welcoming dining space. Eliminate distractions such as television or smartphones, and sit down at a table.

Observe Your Food: Before taking a bite, take a moment to observe your food. Notice the colors, textures, and aromas. Allow yourself to appreciate the effort that went into preparing the meal.

Engage Your Senses: Use all of your senses when you eat. Observe the tastes and sensations in your mouth. Chew slowly and savor each bite.

Listen to Your Body: Become aware of your body's signals of hunger and fullness. Eat when you're hungry and stop when you're satisfied, rather than eating out of habit or until you're uncomfortably full.

Practice Gratitude: Express gratitude for the food you're eating and the nourishment it provides. Consider the path that food takes to get from its source to your plate.

Combining Mindful Eating with Relaxation:
Mindful eating can be enhanced by incorporating relaxation techniques into your meals. This combination not only helps you

appreciate your food but also promotes a sense of calm and well-being. Here's how to integrate relaxation with mindful eating:

Set an Intention: Before your meal, take a moment to set an intention for your eating experience. Express a desire to nourish your body and enjoy your food mindfully.

Deep Breathing: Start your meal with a few deep breaths to calm your nervous system. Take a deep breath, hold it for a short while, and then gently release it.

Gratitude Meditation: Spend a minute in silent reflection or prayer, expressing gratitude for your food, the hands that prepared it, and the nourishment it provides.

Sip Mindfully: If you're drinking a beverage with your meal, take slow sips and savor the flavors. Notice the sensations of warmth or coolness as you sip.

Chew Slowly: As you eat, chew each bite slowly and deliberately. Put your fork down between bites to give yourself time to fully taste and appreciate the food.

Body Scan: During your meal, periodically scan your body for any tension or stress. If you notice areas of tension, take a deep breath and consciously release it.

Silent Meal: Consider having a silent meal, where you eat without conversation or distractions. This allows you to fully immerse yourself in the sensory experience of eating.

Finish with Gratitude: When you finish your meal, express gratitude again for the nourishment you received. Take a moment to reflect on how you feel physically and emotionally.

Benefits of Mindful Eating and Relaxation:

Improved Digestion: Mindful eating can aid digestion by allowing your body to better process and absorb nutrients.

Healthy Weight Management: Eating mindfully can help prevent overeating and make you more attuned to your body's hunger and fullness signals, potentially aiding in weight management.

Reduced Stress: Combining relaxation techniques with mindful eating can reduce stress and anxiety around food, creating a more enjoyable and peaceful mealtime experience.

Enhanced Satisfaction: By savoring each bite, you're likely to find more satisfaction in your meals, which can reduce the desire for unhealthy snacking or emotional eating.

Greater Connection: Mindful eating promotes a deeper connection with your food, fostering an appreciation for the nourishment it provides and the effort that goes into its preparation.

Mindful eating and relaxation are practices that go hand in hand, offering numerous physical, emotional, and spiritual benefits. By bringing mindfulness to your meals and incorporating relaxation techniques, you can transform your relationship with food, promote a sense of well-being, and find joy in every bite.

Yoga and Meditation

Yoga and meditation are time-honored practices that have been revered for their profound impact on physical, mental, and spiritual health. They offer a holistic approach to well-being, promoting not only physical fitness but also emotional balance, mental clarity, and inner peace. In this guide, we'll explore the benefits of yoga and meditation and how you can incorporate them into your daily life.

Yoga: Balancing Mind, Body, and Spirit

Yoga is a comprehensive practice that originated in India over 5,000 years ago. It encompasses various techniques, including physical postures (asanas), breath control (pranayama), meditation, and ethical principles. Here's how yoga can benefit your life:

Physical Fitness: Through a combination of stretching, strengthening, and balance exercises, yoga improves flexibility, enhances muscle tone, and boosts overall physical fitness.

Stress Reduction: Yoga encourages relaxation by calming the nervous system. Regular practice reduces the production of stress hormones like cortisol and promotes a sense of inner peace. [SEP]

Emotional Balance: Yoga helps regulate emotions by encouraging self-awareness and mindfulness. It can reduce anxiety, depression, and mood swings.

Improved Focus: The synchronization of breath and movement in yoga enhances mental concentration and clarity. This can have a positive impact on your work, creativity, and decision-making.

Physical Health: Yoga can alleviate physical ailments such as back pain, arthritis, and hypertension. It also aids in digestion, boosts the immune system, and supports cardiovascular health. [SEP]
Spiritual Growth: For those seeking spiritual growth, yoga provides a path to connect with a higher consciousness or inner self.

Meditation: The Art of Inner Stillness

Meditation is a mental exercise in which you concentrate your attention on a single thing, idea, or task. It's designed to quiet the mind and create a sense of inner stillness. Here's how meditation can benefit your life:

Stress Reduction: Meditation is a potent stress-reduction tool. It helps calm the mind, reduce anxiety, and lower blood pressure.

Emotional Resilience: Regular meditation cultivates emotional resilience by helping you respond to challenging situations with equanimity and poise.

Improved Concentration: Meditation enhances focus and concentration, which can boost productivity and enhance creativity.

Better Sleep: Practicing meditation can improve the quality of your sleep by reducing insomnia and promoting a sense of calm before bedtime.

Enhanced Self-Awareness: Meditation encourages self-reflection, allowing you to better understand your thoughts, emotions, and behaviors.

Spiritual Exploration: For many, meditation is a spiritual practice that fosters a deeper connection with the inner self or a higher power.

How to Get Started:

Choose Your Style: There are various styles of yoga and meditation, each with its unique approach. Explore different practices to find the ones that resonate with you.

Set Aside Time: Dedicate a specific time each day for your practice. Consistency is key to experiencing the full benefits of yoga and meditation.

Seek Guidance: Consider taking classes or finding a qualified instructor to guide you in the early stages of your practice.

Create a Peaceful Space: Designate a quiet, clutter-free space for your practice, whether it's a corner of a room or a serene outdoor spot.

Be Patient: Both yoga and meditation are journeys, not destinations. Be patient with yourself, and allow your practice to evolve over time.

Incorporating yoga and meditation into your daily life can lead to profound positive changes in your physical and mental well-being. These ancient practices offer a sanctuary of inner peace and self-discovery amidst life's hustle and bustle. Whether you seek physical fitness, emotional balance, or spiritual growth, yoga and meditation are powerful tools that can enrich every aspect of your life.

Staying Active and Healthy

Maintaining an active and healthy lifestyle is not just a short-term goal; it's a lifelong commitment to your well-being. Regular physical activity and mindful dietary choices contribute to physical fitness, mental clarity, and overall quality of life. Here's a comprehensive guide to help you stay active and healthy throughout your life.

Physical Activity:

Find Activities You Enjoy: The key to staying active is to engage in activities you love. Whether it's hiking, dancing, swimming, or playing a sport, choose activities that make you excited to move.

Set Realistic Goals: Set achievable fitness goals to keep yourself motivated. These goals can be as simple as taking a daily walk, completing a 5K run, or mastering a challenging yoga pose.

Variety is Key: Avoid monotony by diversifying your physical activities. This not only prevents boredom but also engages different muscle groups and improves overall fitness.

Consistency: Regularity is crucial. Try to get at least 150 minutes a week of moderate-to-intense aerobic activity or 75 minutes of vigorous-to-intense aerobic activity, along with two or more days of muscle-strengthening exercises.

Stay Hydrated: Sufficient hydration is necessary for the best possible physical performance. Before, during, and after exercise, sip water.

Listen to Your Body: Observe the cues your body is sending you. Rest when needed, and don't push yourself too hard to avoid injury.

Warm Up and Cool Down: Begin and end each workout with a warm-up and cool-down period. Stretching helps improve flexibility and reduce the risk of injury.

Healthy Diet:

Balanced Diet: Eat a well-balanced diet full of whole grains, fruits, vegetables, lean meats, and healthy fats. Avoid excessive sugar, processed foods, and saturated fats.

Portion Control: Be mindful of portion sizes to prevent overeating. Use smaller plates to help control portions.

Frequent Meals: Aim for regular, smaller meals throughout the day to maintain stable blood sugar levels and prevent energy dips.

Limit Processed Foods: Limit the amount of processed and fast food you eat because they are frequently heavy in sodium, sugar, and bad fats.

Moderation: Indulge in your favorite treats occasionally, but do so in moderation. Savor the experience, but avoid overindulging.

Stay Hydrated: Water is your best beverage throughout the day. Thirst can occasionally be confused with hunger.

Mental Well-Being:
Stress Management: Practice stress-reduction techniques like meditation, deep breathing, or mindfulness to maintain mental clarity and emotional well-being.

Adequate Sleep: Prioritize sleep as it is essential for mental and physical recovery. Aim for seven to nine hours of good sleep every night.

Social Connections: Nurture meaningful relationships and seek support from friends and family when needed.

Seek Professional Help: If you struggle with mental health issues, do not hesitate to seek help from a mental health professional. It's a sign of strength to ask for assistance.

Lifelong Learning:

Stay Informed: Continuously educate yourself about health and well-being. Stay updated on nutrition, exercise trends, and health-related topics.

Adaptability: Be open to change and adapt your fitness and dietary routines as your body and life circumstances evolve.

Mindful Eating: Practice mindful eating, which involves paying full attention to your food, savoring each bite, and listening to your body's hunger and fullness cues.

Set New Goals: As you age, adjust your fitness and dietary goals to suit your changing needs and capabilities.

Preventive Care: Schedule regular check-ups with healthcare providers for preventive care and early detection of health issues.

Staying active and healthy is an ongoing journey that requires dedication and self-awareness. It's about making choices that prioritize your physical, mental, and emotional well-being. By incorporating these practices into your daily life and embracing them as part of your lifestyle, you can enjoy a long and vibrant journey of health and well-being. Remember that every small step you take today contributes to a healthier and happier future.

Exercise and Physical Activity Tips

Physical activity and exercise are essential for preserving health and wellbeing. Whether you're just starting a fitness journey or looking to enhance your current routine, here are some valuable tips to help you stay active and make the most of your exercise regimen:

1. Set Clear Goals:

Establish specific and achievable fitness goals. Whether it's improving cardiovascular health, building strength, or losing weight, having clear objectives will keep you motivated.

2. Find Activities You Enjoy:

Choose exercises that you genuinely enjoy. This will make it easier to stick with your routine and turn physical activity into a pleasurable part of your life.

3. Mix It Up:

Variety is the spice of life, and it's also essential for a well-rounded fitness routine. Incorporate a combination of aerobic exercises (like walking, running, or swimming), strength training (using weights or resistance bands), and flexibility exercises (such as yoga or stretching).

4. Start Slowly:

If you're new to exercise or returning after a hiatus, begin gradually. Overexertion can lead to injuries or burnout. Start with low-intensity workouts and progressively increase the intensity and duration.

5. Warm Up and Cool Down:
Always warm up your muscles and joints before working out to ensure they are ready for action. Similarly, cool down after your workout to help your body recover gradually.

6. Stay Hydrated:
Drink water before, during, and after your exercise sessions to stay adequately hydrated. Dehydration can impact your performance and health.

7. Proper Form:
Pay attention to your form during exercises. Using the right technique minimizes the chance of damage while also optimizing performance. If you're not sure, think about hiring a certified personal trainer.

8. Listen to Your Body:

Learn to recognize the signals your body sends. If you feel pain, dizziness, or extreme discomfort, stop exercising immediately and seek medical attention if necessary.

9. Consistency Is Key:

Consistency is more important than intensity. Aim for regular exercise, even if it's just a short workout. It's better to maintain a routine than sporadically engage in intense exercise.

10. Rest and Recovery:

In between workouts, give your body time to relax and heal. Fatigue and damage can result from overtraining. Make an effort to take one or two days off each week.

11. Set a Schedule:

Plan your exercise sessions in advance and stick to a schedule. Treat your workouts like important appointments.

12. Exercise with Friends:

Exercising with friends or in a group setting can be motivating and fun. It also provides a sense of accountability.

13. Measure Progress:

Keep track of your progress by recording your workouts, taking measurements, or noting improvements in strength, endurance, or flexibility.

14. Nutrition Matters:

A balanced diet plays a crucial role in your fitness journey. Fuel your body with a combination of carbohydrates, proteins, healthy fats, and vitamins to support your active lifestyle.

15. Consult a Healthcare Professional:

If you have underlying health conditions or are over a certain age, consult with your healthcare provider before starting a new exercise program.

16. Stay Safe Outdoors:

If you exercise outdoors, be mindful of your surroundings. Use sunscreen, wear appropriate clothing and footwear, and be aware of your environment to prevent accidents.

17. Be Patient:

Results take time, so be patient with your progress. Celebrate small victories along the way, and remember that consistency is key to long-term success.

18. Enjoy the Journey:

Exercise isn't just about reaching a destination; it's about enjoying the journey to a healthier, happier you. Enjoy yourself while you go along and embrace the process.

Remember that physical activity isn't solely about achieving a certain look or weight; it's about improving your overall health, boosting your mood, and enhancing your quality of life. By following these tips and adopting a balanced approach to fitness, you can create a sustainable exercise routine that supports your well-being for years to come.

BONUS 21 DAYS MEAL PLAN

Here's a 21-day meal plan that incorporates a variety of nutritious and balanced meals:

Day 1:
Breakfast: Greek yoghurt topped with a honey drizzle and a mixture of berries
Lunch: Grilled chicken Caesar salad
Dinner: Baked salmon with roasted vegetables

Day 2:
Breakfast: Spinach and mushroom omelets
Lunch: Quinoa and avocado salad
Dinner: Turkey and sweet potato casserole

Day 3:
Breakfast: Overnight oats with chia seeds and sliced banana
Lunch: Chicken and rice soup with whole grain bread
Dinner: Veggie and turkey quiche with a side of steamed asparagus

Day 4:

Breakfast: Apple slices and whole grain toast with almond butter

Lunch: Mixed bean salad with a lemon vinaigrette

Dinner: Lentil curry with brown rice

Day 5:

Breakfast: Scrambled eggs with spinach and cherry tomatoes

Lunch: Grilled vegetable wrap with hummus

Dinner: Herbed baked chicken with quinoa and roasted brussels sprouts

Day 6:

Breakfast: Berry and kale smoothie

Lunch: Tuna salad with mixed greens

Dinner: Grilled prawns and marinara sauce over zucchini noodles

Day 7:

Breakfast: Oatmeal with sliced peaches and a sprinkle of almonds

Lunch: Balsamic glaze and fresh basil on a caprese salad

Dinner: Teriyaki tofu stir-fry with broccoli and brown rice

Day 8:

Breakfast: Greek yoghurt topped with mixed berries on whole grain waffles

Lunch: Chickpea salad with cucumber, bell peppers, and a lemon-tahini dressing

Dinner: Baked cod with quinoa pilaf and steamed green beans

Day 9:

Breakfast: Chia seed pudding with sliced mango and a sprinkle of nuts

Lunch: Spinach and feta stuffed bell peppers

Dinner: Lentil and vegetable curry served with whole wheat naan

Day 10:

Breakfast: Poached eggs, cherry tomatoes, and avocado toast

Lunch: Grilled chicken and vegetable skewers with a side of quinoa

Dinner: Mushroom risotto with a side salad

Day 11:

Breakfast: Banana and almond butter smoothie

Lunch: Tuna and white bean salad with lemon-dill dressing

Dinner: Baked sweet potatoes with black bean and corn salsa

Day 12:

Breakfast: Greek yogurt parfait with granola and sliced strawberries

Lunch: Bell peppers filled with quinoa and black beans

Dinner: Grilled teriyaki chicken with stir-fried vegetables and brown rice

Day 13:

Breakfast: Scrambled tofu with sautéed spinach and whole grain toast

Lunch: Mixed greens salad with grilled tofu and a citrus vinaigrette

Dinner: Spaghetti squash with marinara sauce and turkey meatballs

Day 14:

Breakfast: Blueberry and spinach smoothie

Lunch: Caprese quinoa salad with fresh basil and balsamic glaze

Dinner: Baked lemon herb tilapia with quinoa and roasted asparagus

Day 15:

Breakfast: Pancakes made with whole grains, fresh fruit, and honey drizzled over them

Lunch: Chicken and vegetable kebabs with a side of tabbouleh

Dinner: Veggie-packed lentil soup with a side of whole grain bread

Day 16:

Breakfast: Acai bowl topped with granola, coconut, and mixed berries

Lunch: Quinoa and kale salad with roasted chickpeas and a lemon tahini dressing

Dinner: Grilled shrimp tacos with cabbage slaw and avocado

Day 17:

Breakfast: Cottage cheese with sliced peaches and a sprinkle of nuts

Lunch: Caprese quinoa stuffed bell peppers

Dinner: Baked chicken with sweet potato wedges and a side of steamed broccoli

Day 18:

Breakfast: Fruit and nut muesli with almond milk

Lunch: Lentil salad with mixed greens and a balsamic vinaigrette

Dinner: Tofu and vegetable stir-fry with brown rice

Day 19:

Breakfast: Whole grain toast with smoked salmon and avocado

Lunch: Spinach and chickpea curry with quinoa

Dinner: Turkey and vegetable skewers with herbed couscous

Day 20:

Breakfast: Greek yoghurt topped with honeydew and sliced bananas

Lunch: Mediterranean quinoa salad with olives and feta cheese

Dinner: Baked cod with a side of wild rice and roasted vegetables

Day 21:

Breakfast: Omelette with tomatoes, spinach, and feta cheese

Lunch: Chickpea and vegetable wrap with hummus

Dinner: Grilled steak with sweet potato mash and grilled asparagus

Feel free to mix and match these meal ideas throughout the 21 days to keep your meals varied and satisfying. Adjust portion sizes to suit your individual needs and consider any dietary preferences or restrictions you might have while following this plan.

Printed in Great Britain
by Amazon

41577849R00175